D0743459

Thyroid Cancer for Beginners

Glenda Shepherd

authorHOUSE®

AuthorHouse™ UK Ltd.
500 Avebury Boulevard
Central Milton Keynes, MK9 2BE
www.authorhouse.co.uk
Phone: 08001974150

© 2009 Glenda Shepherd. All rights reserved.

No part of this book may be reproduced, stored in a retrieval system, or transmitted by any means without the written permission of the author.

First published by AuthorHouse 4/7/2009

ISBN: 978-1-4389-6583-3 (sc)

ISBN: 978-1-4389-6583-3

Printed in the United States of America
Bloomington, Indiana

This book is printed on acid-free paper.

Dedicated to my husband Phil, who has given me unconditional love and support in the darkest times, and to the Surgeons, Oncologist and Healer whose treatments between them have increased my lifespan.

INTRODUCTION

Thyroid cancer is an unusual cancer, but fortunately often a very treatable one. Nobody really knows what causes it. As it affects mostly women, one theory is that the sudden weight gain and weight loss during pregnancy precipitates it, but there is also the theory that radiation to the face and neck during childhood (for example dental x-rays) may be a factor, and also some say the fallout from Chernobyl could be a cause. Incidences are rising. GP's only get to see one or two cases per year, so they are not always very knowledgeable on treatment procedures. Anyone newly-diagnosed with thyroid cancer will find only some specialist hospitals can treat it (for example the hospital where I work does not treat it, and the Oncologist there does not know much about it). They will also find that treatment procedures vary up and down the country. In some areas patients are offered multiple radioactive Iodine (RAI) treatments, but patients in other areas are not. Some patients are given tracer scans with a very low dose of radioactive Iodine before treatment is given, to see whether there is any uptake of radiation in the thyroid tissue, so in theory making sure that the thyroid tissue is receptive to the larger dose of radiation to come. Others are not offered a tracer scan, as another theory is that it stuns the thyroid cells and does not make them as receptive to the actual therapeutic dose of RAI and prolongs the treatment.

There can also be differences of opinion on how long a patient is left on the T3 fast-acting Liothyronine Sodium before he or she is given the slower-releasing T4 Levothyroxine tablets that they will take for life. I have discovered this by joining the internet site www.thyroidcancersupportuk.org   Ordinary people just like me are comparing treatment procedures and waiting times for treatment which vary enormously according to where they live. Join the site and you will find a wealth of information and friendly helpful people, all fellow-sufferers. They may not always have the same opinions as yourself, but will be interested in hearing what you have to say regarding your treatment and commenting on it.

I hope this book is informative for anyone newly-diagnosed with thyroid cancer. I suppose we have the 'best' sort of cancer you can get, as survival rates are usually around 95%. I have heard it said that thyroid cancer is not really a cancer, but it will certainly prove fatal if not treated as there will probably be spread to the lungs and/or bones.

They say everyone has a story to tell. I didn't for a moment expect mine would be this one.

Glenda Shepherd (December 2008)

Contents

CHAPTER ONE – THE START OF IT ALL

On the Isle of Wight's Sandown beach in October 2004, I stand barefoot with my husband, Phil, at the water's edge. Looking back across the beach, I spot Phil's sister Mary and her husband Dave wrapped up in towels on their sunbeds to protect them from the cold wind that has suddenly sprung up. Dave and his camera are never too far away from each other, and I hear him calling to us to pose for a photo. He walks over to us, camera in hand, and says something silly to make us laugh whilst he snaps away. The four of us are on a long weekend break staying at a bungalow in Bembridge owned by Dave's sister Betty. We'd all had a pretty good year so far. We had attended the wedding of our eldest son Lee to Sarah on a glorious day in May, and Mary and Dave had recently announced a third grandchild was on the way. Phil and I were due to become grandparents the following July as Sarah was now newly pregnant. We were also looking forward to another long weekend break together at the Center Parcs holiday village in Elveden, Suffolk, in December, about a half hour drive from our home. The short break would not only be with Mary, Dave and their daughter Jenny, but also Lee and Sarah were coming along and our youngest son Matthew and his girlfriend Anna. We often met up with Mary and Dave, and we had all married within a week of each other early in October 1980. We had originally lived near to them in Croydon, Surrey, where Phil had been born and brought up, but had moved to a village near Bury St Edmunds in 1991 due to Phil's new job being based in Palgrave, near Diss in Norfolk. Problems had arisen when it was taking him three hours to travel to Palgrave from Croydon, and usually longer than that to travel home every night. We had two young sons and welcomed taking them out of the London suburbs and living the country life. After the first year of adjustment to the slower pace of life we were now fully-fledged country folk. After 13 years of living the country life, we had no plans to ever move back to London.

What we were all unaware of as we posed for the photo on Sandown beach, was that before a month had gone by Dave was to suffer a heart attack (which luckily he recovered from after treatment), and I was to find a lump in my neck whilst putting on a necklace. Nobody knows what fate has in store. I read somewhere that the world was made round so we don't see too far down the road. Perhaps that's just as well.

I had no idea how long the lump had been there. The Oncologist I saw a few months into the treatment said it could have been there for years. The neck area is not a place where you're told to check for lumps. Leaflets picked up in the GP surgery told me that I needed to be 'breast aware' and to have cervical smears every three years, but I'd never even considered the neck area when thinking about cancer – even though I've since found out that thyroid cancer affects mostly women. My father and his brother had both died of cancer at age 49, one of prostate cancer and the other of a brain tumour. My mother contracted cancer of the uterus in her sixties, but survived after having a hysterectomy and radiotherapy (she is now in her eighties and living near me in warden-assisted sheltered housing). Two of my grandparents had also died in their seventies of cancer, one of pancreatic cancer, and the other of lung cancer (probably due to my grandfather being a heavy smoker though). As I had approached my forties I started to worry that maybe I too was at risk of cancer due to this unhealthy legacy. Also over the previous decade I had begun to put on weight and suffered with terrible PMT symptoms. At about age 37 I was feeling so awful that I had to do something about it. I saw a Gynaecologist who prescribed the mini-pill (Norethisterone) which miraculously took all my PMT symptoms away, and I began a long-overdue exercise programme. Ten years on, at age 47, I was still jogging nearly every day before starting work at 7.30am as a Ward Clerk at a local hospital, rising at 5.15am to run a 2-mile circuit of our picturesque village. I enjoyed the early morning sunrises and the feeling that the village was mine alone as I pounded the pavements when everyone else was in bed. I ate a low-fat diet to keep my weight down; indeed since being pregnant with Matthew in 1985 I could not stomach any fried or fatty foods anyway, they would instantly make me feel nauseous. In my early forties I had also started to feel sick if I had cows milk in tea (a skin test confirmed a milk intolerance), and cheese and chocolate which previously I had eaten with abandon started off migraines, so I had switched to Soya milk, which luckily I preferred the taste of in tea (de-caffeinated of course!). From being overweight and feeling miserable and eating lots of unhealthy foods in my thirties, I was now the veritable picture of health. The only problem I had suffered with during the past couple of years was a locking jaw at night. I had no idea why the jaw locked whilst I was asleep – the Dentist said that it could be caused by the unconscious grinding of my teeth.

I decided to make an appointment with the GP about the lump in my neck but was not overly worried. It was probably a pulled muscle due to all the neck exercises I did to keep the ravages of time at bay.

The end of November 2004 saw me waiting in the GP surgery. The Doctor felt my neck and noted that the lump moved when I swallowed. She wanted to refer me to a Consultant Endocrinologist at the hospital where I worked, as she thought I had a cyst on my thyroid. The thyroid is a butterfly-shaped gland at the front of the neck which secretes the hormone Thyroxine, and this has an effect on the body's metabolic rate (how quickly you burn up food). As I was included on Phil's medical insurance policy and wanted to be seen sooner rather than later, I let the GP know I would like to be seen privately at the Nuffield hospital in Bury St Edmunds. I completed the paperwork required and waited for an appointment to arrive through the post.

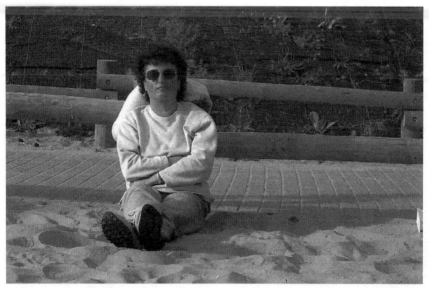

The lump seems quite visible here on a Center Parcs holiday in August 2003, but surprisingly enough I never noticed it until over a year later.

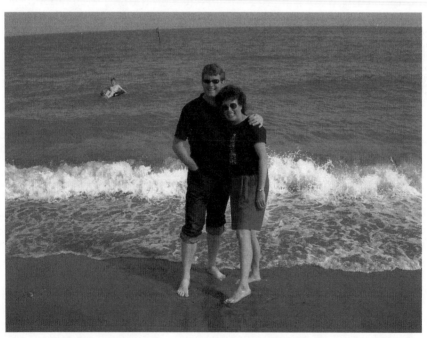

Photo shows Phil and I on the beach at Sandown, Isle of Wight. October 2004. Dave's saying something to make us laugh, but I can't remember what.

CHAPTER TWO – EARLY YEARS

I was born Glenda Ann Wood on October 28th 1957 in East London, and spent my early childhood living in the East London suburb of Poplar, with my parents. Originally we had lived in a large (and haunted) flat above what used to be Barclays Bank at 819 Commercial Road (the flat is still there, but the bank is now a café). I was aware at a very young age of a strange presence there; my bedroom was always colder than the rest of the house, and I often saw the ghosts of animals in the flat. My mother once told me of an occasion where I was staying overnight with my grandmother, but the imprint of a body in my bed still remained even though the bed had been tidied that morning. I remember as a very young child that sometimes my bed would shake uncontrollably and I would dive under the covers in fright, hoping the shaking would go away. I had no idea what caused it, and over a period of time accepted it as 'normal'. The psychic phenomena I experienced as a young child in the flat started my lifelong interest in the spirit world. My parents rented the flat at a reduced rate as my father was a bank employee (or maybe it was cheap because of the other-wordly presence?). Years later I found out that somebody had committed suicide in the flat. It was no place for a young child of five to live in though, as there were no children nearby to play with, and I was too young and the streets below far too busy for me to play outside. I had no siblings, and had started to play with imaginary friends. My parents wanted a home in a quieter location away from the constant heavy traffic rumbling past outside, and from the undesirables that often slept on the main doorstep downstairs that led out onto the Commercial Road. They also wanted to move me from Mayflower Primary School in Upper North Street, as I was not enjoying the experience (to put it mildly). The council found us a prefabricated home a mile or so away at number 3 Layfield Place (off Byron Street, but alas no longer there) that was supposed to have been only temporary whilst we waited for permanent accommodation. The 'temporary' wait eventually stretched to seven years!

The 'prefab' as far as I was concerned was idyllic. I much preferred it to the flat in Commercial Road, as we were on the ground floor and I could play in our sizeable garden. The psychic happenings disappeared, and were only to surface very infrequently from then on. I found a couple of 'best' friends who lived nearby, and attended a new school, Manorfield Primary, in St. Leonard's road, where my fledgling musical talents were encouraged by the formidable Miss Anderson . I began to play the violin, but the road to perfection was long (after an evening sawing away, I found that Dad had 'accidentally' trodden on the violin the next morning!). At age 11 I attended George Green Grammar School in the East India Dock Road. My fondest memories of that school were throwing left-overs from my lunch down to the boys' playground on street level from the girls' playground up on the roof, and hoping to score a direct hit on one of the more obnoxious boys in the process who constantly made fun of my curly hair. When going home from school I had to walk through Crisp Street with all its shops and market stalls, and I can still hear all the market traders' calls in my head. My favourite stall was the old 45rpm record stall. Most of my pocket money was blown on Rock n' Roll records, comics, sweets, and Enid Blyton books bought from Segal's bookshop (my favourite shop) on the East India Dock Road .

My childhood years were very happy and I had total freedom to roam the streets with friends, something I would not have let my own children do if they had been brought up in the same part of London today, as it has now totally changed as you can imagine. We explored condemned houses that were due to be demolished to make way for the A102M motorway, played 'Knock Down Ginger' in Balfron Towers, and scared ourselves silly playing 'Chicken' down by the Blackwall Tunnel. Mum and Dad were not on the end of a mobile phone, and if we got into scrapes, then we had to get out of them ourselves. When our prefab home (and in fact Layfield Place itself) was due to be demolished to make way for what is now a technical college, the council had no choice but to re-house us. We moved across the river and I suddenly had to leave behind all that was familiar when I was 13.

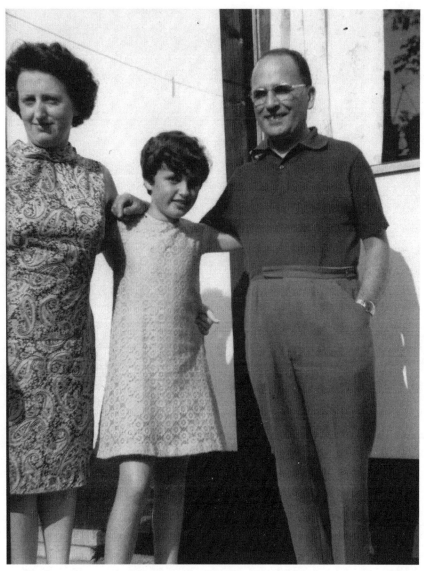

Aged about 10 with my parents outside our prefab home in Poplar in the Sixties'.

My teenage years were spent living in Kidbrooke, South East London, on a huge sprawling council estate that is now thankfully in the process of being demolished. I loathed the estate as soon as I saw it, and my opinion never changed in the seven or so years that I lived there. I was content though with my new school, Kidbrooke Comprehensive (the same school that latterly Jamie Oliver trialled with the new healthy school meals), after the initial strangeness had worn off. I had a few very good friends, and took part with them in virtually all extra-curricular musical activities. I left school in 1976 and went to work as a Laboratory Technician for a company that has now been taken over by GlaxoSmithKline. The following year, when I was 19, my father died of cancer of the prostate which had spread to his bones. He had contracted cancer at the age of 47; the same age as I had been when I found the lump in my neck. I helped my mother to organise his funeral, but due to my young age I realise with hindsight that I was not much of a comfort to her in the months afterwards.

I knew by the age of 20 that I wanted to leave home to forge a life of my own, as my late nights (due to my regular attendance at various local discotheques) were having an unfortunate effect on my mother's sleeping habits (what goes around comes around, and it would be me waiting at the top of the stairs 25 years later as Lee crept up at 4am after a night out on the lash). I rented a flat in Anerley near Crystal Palace with a workmate. It certainly helped both of us as my mother then aged 54, after finding herself living alone for the first time in 25 years, learned to drive, drove herself and friends to various local dances, and even in time found a boyfriend. I quickly learnt to look after myself, cook, and do small repair jobs on my car. Myself and my flatmate had the time of our lives whilst living in our little attic flat, staying out dancing until late, giving parties, and falling in love with undesirable work colleagues, all the things you do when you're young and silly!

Whilst living at the flat in Anerley, I met the man who was to be my husband. Phil had also come from a huge council estate in New Addington, Croydon and had lots of siblings, something I envied him for, having always wanted a sister or brother of my own. We became engaged three months after meeting, and married on October 11th 1980 in St. James Church, Kidbrooke. In the same month I left my job due to various allergies to workplace conditions, and became a Library Assistant at Anerley library near to my old attic flat in Waldegrave Road. We went on to have two sons, Lee, born in July 1982, and Matthew, born in November 1985. Life was good. I had a lovely husband, two sons to love and care for, and we now had a home of our own in Addiscome near Croydon, albeit with a mortgage up to the hilt. I stayed at home for 12 years looking after the boys, which had its rewards as well as its down moments. During that time we moved from London to a village near Bury St Edmunds to be closer to Phil's workplace, and also to give the boys a better life. When Lee was 12 and Matthew was 8 I started back at work as an Office Clerk for a small company dealing in the sales of lime and fertiliser to the farmer. It had taken me three years of applying for jobs to secure the post, and I was beginning to think that at the age of 36 and with two young children I would never work again. I am very determined though, and vowed I would not give up until I did get a job. I carried on over the next 10 years through two other administration jobs ending up working as a Ward Clerk at my local hospital in Bury St Edmunds, and all the time applying for higher-grade administration vacancies in the NHS which sadly seemed very elusive. I did not mind working as a Ward Clerk though, but was ever hopeful that something better would be just around the corner. Unfortunately it would be something worse around the corner and it was coming straight at me.............

CHAPTER THREE – VISIT TO THE ENDOCRINOLOGIST & 1ST SCAN

The appointment date to see the Consultant Endocrinologist was not long in arriving. I went to see him in early December 2004 at his private clinic at the Nuffield hospital. He explained that the lump probably was a cyst, but would take some blood to check if the thyroid was working properly, and there would be more blood tests and a 24-hour urine test also to determine whether cancer was present, but he stressed that the lump probably wasn't cancerous at all as there was no history of thyroid cancer in my family. I was told that I would also need an ultrasound scan and possibly a needle biopsy of the cyst at the same time. I explained I would soon be on a long weekend break at Center Parcs and he said he would speak to the Consultant Radiologist to ensure I had the scan before I went. He said it was also a good idea to get a sample of blood to see if I was at the menopause. I was to come back and see him near the end of December for the results. His Nurse took the blood tests there and then, and I was sent home with two large plastic urine collection bottles. He explained that as I was at work during the week, it would be best to wait for a Sunday to fill the urine bottles as it would be more convenient than having to carry them about at work all day! I agreed totally, and spent the next Sunday dutifully filling the bottles ready to take to Pathology on the Monday morning when I went back to work. We were due for our Center Parcs visit on the 10th December and on the 9th I had my ultrasound scan in the X-Ray Department at the Nuffield. The Consultant Radiologist could see my thyroid was covered in cysts. He said he wasn't worried as the whole thyroid was lumpy rather than just one piece of it. He said he wasn't even going to take a needle biopsy, as the result would just come back as benign cells. I was reassured when he said nothing needed to be done other than regular check-ups to see if the cyst had grown any bigger. He would report back to the Endocrinologist and I would get his report and the results of the blood tests when I had my second endocrinology appointment just before Christmas. He thought it was a multinodular goitre (looking back with hindsight, it would have been a good idea at that point to seek a second opinion!).

Meanwhile there was Center Parcs to enjoy. Myself and Phil, Lee now aged 22 and his new wife Sarah, plus Matthew aged 19 and girlfriend Anna met up with Mary, Dave, and Jenny. We had adjoining chalets and everyone was set to have a good time. We had all been visiting Center Parcs since the boys and Jenny were small. Dave had recently had to have one of his arteries opened up with a stent. The artery had become clogged over the years, which had given him the mild heart attack a couple of months before. He looked pale and seemed more tired than usual, but was still cracking jokes and making people laugh. He didn't fancy playing Badminton which he had done in the past (which was a shame as he's so bad at it that it's hysterical to watch), but to my surprise put on a pair of roller skates and skated around the rink with the rest of us. We couldn't believe he'd been in the Coronary Care Unit only a short while before, and now here he was balancing on a pair of skates. He'd had to change his diet to a low-fat one which meant cutting out his beloved cheese, but other than that was set to lead a normal life.

Center Parcs turned out to be not so much fun as it had been in previous years when the boys and Jenny were small. I was still thinking about the lump in my neck and what the blood tests would reveal. Dave was tired and not as jolly as he used to be (understandable due to what he'd undergone), and there was also some friction between a few of the young people, which also affected us and Mary and Dave. Unhappily the holiday ended on a rather sour note, and I think everyone was pleased to go home on the last day.

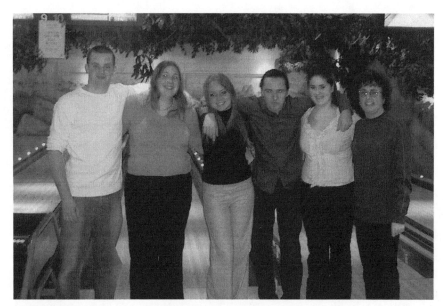

Left to right, Lee, Sarah, Jenny, Matt, Anna, and myself at Center Parcs Dec 04

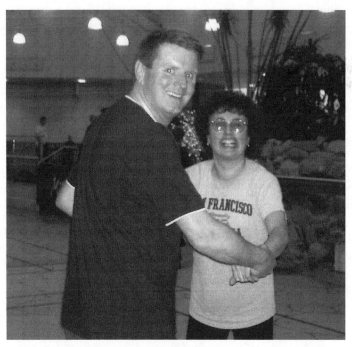

Phil and I skating at Center Parcs December 2004.

A week or so after the Center Parcs break, it was time to return to the Endocrinologist at the Nuffield hospital to learn the results of all the tests. He was most encouraging. He told me my thyroid was working normally, that the blood and urine tests were clear – indeed I had lovely 'rich' blood. He diagnosed a multinodular goitre (I suppose he was basing his findings on the ultrasound report) and told me I would need only regular scans to keep an eye on the cyst to check it wasn't getting any bigger. If it wasn't causing me any problems he suggested leaving it alone. The only cloud on the horizon was that he was unable to determine if I was menopausal. Apparently the Norethisterone tablets which I had been taking for ten years to combat the dreadful symptoms of pre-menstrual tension were keeping my follicle stimulating hormone and luteinising hormone levels artificially low (if I had been menopausal the levels would have been sky-high). In order to obtain a blood sample that wasn't affected by the tablets, I would have to come off them for at least three months and then have another blood test. I could do that I thought – that was easy. What with my healthy eating I probably wouldn't have the symptoms now anyway. I made an appointment for March 29th to have another check-up scan and then I positively skipped out of the hospital – now I could enjoy Christmas with my family.

We usually treat ourselves and have Christmas day lunch out at a restaurant. That year it was at the Rushbrooke Arms in Bury St Edmunds with Phil, Matt, Anna and my mother. A New Year's Eve dinner and dance at The Quality Hotel in Norwich was planned with Phil, Lee and Sarah (ever-expanding with our first grandchild), and Matt and Anna. We stayed overnight at the hotel and all had an enjoyable time. We usually saw Mary and Dave over the Christmas period but this year they had other plans (I think the disappointing Center Parcs holiday still loomed large in everyone's minds).

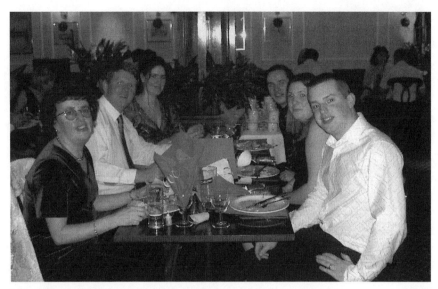

New Year's Eve dinner at The Quality Hotel, Norwich.
Left side from the front, myself, Phil, and Anna. Right side from the front, Lee, Sarah, and Matt.

CHAPTER FOUR – VISIT TO THE ENDOCRINOLOGIST & 2ND SCAN

January and February 2005 passed in the usual whirlwind of work, eat, and sleep. I was also organising quite a few gigs for Matt's Heavy Rock band and we were often out weekends until the early hours at gigs in London and the South East. Phil and I had grown up in the Seventies' listening to loud Rock bands, and it was with a certain amount of relief when Matt mastered the intricacies of the electric guitar and veered towards the music we loved instead of the (as far as I'm concerned) terrible House, Garage, Trance, Dance, Rap/crap genres that Lee favoured as a teenager and had us reaching in the past for the earplugs. Funnily enough though, as Lee has got older he plays Rock music in his van all day, so perhaps some of our tastes did rub off on him after all.

I kept a close watch on the cyst during January and February to see if it was getting any bigger. Towards the end of February I thought that it had increased in size a little bit, but decided the scan in March would show if it had. I felt ok. I'd had no real PMT symptoms either. Thank goodness I can come off the tablets now I thought, because it must be the healthy eating that had altered my body chemistry.

By the time the scan was due at the end of March, I knew the cyst was bigger. I could feel it in my neck as it started to cause a little pressure. I was often getting choking feelings and had to keep coughing, especially if I laid on my left side. I mentioned all this to the Radiologist who again performed the scan, and he said it had increased only marginally. I mentioned it again at the next appointment with the Endocrinologist on April 11th where I was to be told the result of the latest scan. He surprisingly said that although the Radiologist had told him verbally that the cyst was bigger, he hadn't actually written the fact on his report. The Endocrinologist asked me what I wanted to do about the cyst. He said if it continued growing, it would possibly interfere with my swallowing and breathing mechanisms. I had already decided upon surgery to remove it before the appointment, after having had a surprise telephone conversation with my aunt a week or so previously. The end result being I was to be referred to a Consultant Endocrine Surgeon who would surgically remove the cyst at the Nuffield in Bury St Edmunds in the near future.

I had found out, whilst speaking on the phone to my aunt in March, that she had had a cyst on her thyroid removed about ten years previously. I hadn't been aware of this, as we did not see each other very often. She had told me her cyst had been the size of a fist and had spread down into her chest, but had not been cancerous. Doctors had taken half of her thyroid gland away in order to remove the cyst, but apart from recently having to start taking Thyroxine tablets because of excessive tiredness, she was now feeling fine. She also thought her own mother had had thyroid problems which were never treated during her lifetime. I realised that thyroid disease probably ran in my father's side of the family and I seemed to have inherited this onerous trait. Oh well, I mused, I'll just have to get by with half my thyroid, a small price to pay for ridding my body of the cyst.

The Endocrinologist also asked how it had been for me coming off the Norethisterone tablets in December. I mentioned the two symptom-free periods which occurred in January and February, but so far at the end of March no period had arrived. He said it was common to miss periods when coming off long-term use of hormone tablets.

My periods still hadn't returned by May 3rd, the date of the Surgeon's appointment. I wondered how long I would have waited on the NHS to be seen, and thanked my lucky stars that I was covered by medical insurance. I sat and faced the Surgeon on that Tuesday morning, and he explained that it was too dangerous to undertake a partial thyroidectomy. If in later years the remaining thyroid gland also needed to be removed, there would have been too much scar tissue in place from the first operation, and the Surgeon would have had trouble seeing what he was doing with this in the way. He told me that the operation would be a total thyroidectomy and that it was a major operation, possibly taking about three hours to perform. His duty was also to tell me of the possible damage to the nerves controlling the vocal cords as he would have to be working quite near the voice box, and of the inadvertent removal of the parathyroid glands during the operation, which control Calcium metabolism. He reassured me that he was experienced at thyroid removals and his patients did not often suffer these consequences, but it was his duty to ensure I was fully informed of the dangers involved. He reassured me that he always took pains to find and trace the nerve to the voice box before removing the thyroid, and blood tests were taken soon after surgery to check the blood Calcium levels which would start to drop if the parathyroid glands had been caught up in the removed thyroid tissue.

I decided I had no choice but to go ahead with the surgery. I realised the Anaesthetist might have a problem with my locking jaw when he put me to sleep and tried to put the intubation tube down my throat to ventilate me before surgery. I mentioned this to the Surgeon who said he would refer me to a Consultant Oral Surgeon. I had never seen so many doctors in my life in the space of just a few months. All I had ever had were colds and coughs and the usual childhood illnesses, and now I was facing a major operation and possibly another one on my locking jaw.

On the next page are the original ultrasound scan reports showing that the Radiologist felt no biopsy was needed as only an 'intra-cystic papilloma' (benign tumour) might possibly be found, and that on the second scan he had failed to mention the enlargement that had taken place. He had however mentioned it verbally to the Endocrinologist.

Our Ref: RPB/AKB

23rd November 2004

Dr
The Bury St Edmunds Nuffield Hospital
St Marys Square
Bury St Edmunds
Suffolk
IP33 2AA

Dear Dr

Glenda Shepherd DOB 28.10.1957

ULTRASOUND THYROID   23.11.04   Reported 23.11.04

Both lobes of the thyroid show diffuse focal nodular change with cystic areas within. On the right side there is a relatively well defined cyst of approximately 5 mms with an obvious echogenic centre. The nature of this is unclear and may represent an old haemorrhage but obviously an intra-cystic papilloma cannot be excluded.   The nodular change throughout the remainder of the right lobe of thyroid is evident. Within the left lobe in the upper pole there is extensive nodular change with obvious calcification within. In the lower pole on the left side extending into the isthmus there is some cystic areas. This would appear to be the palpable area.

In light of the above I think needling the lower aspect is not indicated and I think possibly trying to needle the right cystic lesion would be extremely difficult. Can we discuss with regard to further assessment?

Dr

29th March 2005

Consultant Physician
The Bury St Edmunds Nuffield Hospital
St Marys Square
Bury St Edmunds
Suffolk
IP33 2AA

Dear Dr

Glenda Shepherd DOB 28.10.1957

ULTRASOUND THYROID   29.03.05   Reported 29.03.05

The multi nodular changes around both lobes of the thyroid are again noted. I think there has been little significant change from previous examination. Could we please discuss further assessment?

Dr

CHAPTER FIVE – APPOINTMENT WITH THE ORAL SURGEON

A couple of weeks after the appointment with the Surgeon, I received a letter from the Nuffield hospital to say the date for my surgery was Monday June 13th 2005 and I needed to attend the Pre-Admission Clinic on June 2nd. There was also an appointment for me to see the Oral Surgeon on June 7th for my jaw problems. Bliss and joy. The Pre-Admission Nurse was kindness personified. I had nose and groin swabs to check I was not MRSA positive. As I worked in an NHS hospital, they were particularly worried about this, as the patients in the Nuffield all had their own rooms and MRSA was unheard of. I had my blood pressure and heart rate checked, which because I was nervous was running a little high (I had begun to suffer from chronic white-coat syndrome!). The in-house Doctor took some blood, listened to my heart, asked me if I had any cracked teeth, and gave me an ECG which showed no problems. I mentioned a crack in a lower molar which caused pain if I chewed on any hard foodstuffs. The pain had been there for about 5 years and caused only intermittent problems, and the Dentist had suggested leaving it alone. My temperature was normal. I had started a very heavy period on May 20th which was in its 14th day with no sign of stopping, so did not want to do a urine test. The Nurse said not to worry as that could be done on the day of admission. I secretly hoped the period would be finished before then, as I didn't really want to have to cope with that as well. I made a mental note to give it one more month to see if things settled down and then resume the Norethisterone tablets if the periods were still haywire. I mentioned the locking jaw dysfunction, and the Doctor said it could be a problem during the operation and he made a note of it.

I was starting to feel nervous about the operation. I had never had an anaesthetic or any sort of operation before. I had only been in hospital twice before, and each time had come out holding a baby. That wasn't going to happen this time. I wondered what the Oral Surgeon would say about the locking jaw. Perhaps he would stop the operation from going ahead.

The Maxillo-facial (Oral) Surgeon felt all around my jaw and asked me to open and close my mouth. My mouth apparently pulled down to the right. He said the jaw was out of alignment, and he then sent me for an x-ray which revealed quite a bit of wear and tear on the left jaw joint, probably due to grinding my teeth whilst asleep. The result was I would need surgery to repair the left side of the jaw, but the operation on my thyroid could go ahead – the Anaesthetist would just need to be careful when manipulating it. Meanwhile he said he would write to my Dentist to instruct him to make me a night-time splint, which would solve the locking problem in the short-term. I knew I would never be able to sleep with any sort of device in my mouth, so discounted that solution immediately. He told me to make another appointment to see him when I wanted the surgery done. From 47 years with no medical problems to two operations needed probably only a few months apart, all my Christmases had come at once.

CHAPTER SIX - THE DAY OF THE THYROIDECTOMY

Phil drove me to the Nuffield hospital on the day of surgery. I likened it mentally to a drive to the executioner's chamber. I'd had nothing to eat or drink as requested and was feeling terribly nervous. My work colleagues had all wished me well and the Ward Manager had given me three weeks off to recuperate. I hoped that was all I needed.

I was shown to room 26 - a pleasant downstairs room with its own bath and toilet, and patio doors leading on to a communal garden. There was the usual hospital bed and call bells, but also carpet on the floor, an armchair, television, and chairs for visitors. Phil and I were told by a Nurse that I was on the afternoon list for surgery, and during the morning would be seen by the in-house Doctor and Anaesthetist. I was disappointed to have to wait at least another five hours before surgery. I was feeling tired and shaky, through lack of sleep and food, and wanted it to be over with quickly. I was given menus to fill out for supper that night, and the following day's meals. The food sounded quite nice and I was eager to eat some of it. I mentioned that I did not eat dairy produce to the 'Hostess' who came to collect the menus and she said that would not be a problem. The Chef could make my usual morning porridge with Soya milk.

We settled down resigned to the long wait. I tried to concentrate on a crossword puzzle book I had brought in and Phil read the morning newspaper. Over the next few years he would become quite an expert at sitting in hospital rooms (a sixth sense told him what I required when I was wheeled back from various operations), but this was his first time as my little helper, apart from when I had had babies over 20 years previously. I couldn't settle and opened the patio doors to go into the garden. It was peaceful – all the other patients were still in bed I assumed, and for a while watched the birds feeding on the bird table. I went into the bathroom and rinsed my mouth several times for something to do. The temptation to take a giant swig of water was almost too much. Phil wouldn't eat or drink anything in front of me, so he stayed nil by mouth too.

We were left to our own devices for almost four hours. Towards lunchtime the Anaesthetist came in. He listened to my chest, asked if I was allergic to any medications and if I had had a bad reaction in the past to any anaesthetics. I replied I knew of no medications I was allergic to, and that I had never had an anaesthetic before. I told him of the locking jaw problem and he noted it on the pink anaesthetic card. He told me I looked nervous and I assured him I was terrified.

Things started to move a bit after that. The Doctor came in and prescribed some tranquilisers to settle me as he'd obviously communicated with the Anaesthetist. The Nurse put an ID wristband on me, measured me for stockings to combat DVT (blood clots forming in the legs due to being immobile), and told me to put on my hospital gown. Phil tied it up at the back and assured me my behind was not hanging out. Nurse came back with the stockings and put them on for me. They felt quite tight and she said they were very good at stopping blood clots forming, and that I could take them home afterwards to use on any long-haul airplane flight. We had a Caribbean cruise booked in November to celebrate our 25th wedding anniversary and I resolved to use them again then. Nurse gave me the medications the Doctor had prescribed and also a pre-med to make me feel sleepy. I was told to get into bed, which I dutifully did. I stared at the ceiling and prayed for sleep but it did not come. Suddenly there was panic – Nurse appeared again and asked had I signed a consent form? I replied in the negative. Organised chaos ensued as the Surgeon had to be found to give me the consent form and I had just been given heavy medication. A few moments later he appeared with the form for signing. I was still lucid when I signed it and still fully awake when the Porter came to take me to the operating theatre just before 2 o'clock. Phil walked down with me, gave me a kiss, and said he would see me later. He probably then went off for some well deserved lunch.

The Anaesthetist greeted me inside the theatre, checked my wristband against his operating list and began to put a cannula in my left hand.

He good-naturedly complained that ladies' veins were always smaller. He then injected a liquid into the cannula and said it would make me feel sleepy. It certainly did, as I remember nothing after that until I woke up in the Recovery Room some three hours later. I was in a sitting position propped up with pillows instead of lying down, and the Recovery Room Nurse assured me that now I was awake, I could be taken back to my room.

CHAPTER SEVEN – THE AFTERMATH OF THE THYROIDECTOMY

Feeling much relieved that it was all over, I was wheeled back to room 26. There was Phil sitting waiting patiently to tend to my every need, bless him. I felt wide awake and not at all sick. I'd heard the usual tales of patients being sick after surgery and resigned myself to the fact that it would probably happen to me. The Anaesthetist had told me on his earlier visit that he always gave his patients a powerful anti-sickness drug through the cannula and I was pleased to say it was still working. There were devices on my lower legs that inflated and deflated at regular intervals, obviously helping out the stockings in their anti-DVT mission, and an oxygen tube going into my nose to oxygenate my red blood cells I was told.

I reached up to feel my neck but Phil gently took my arm and said not to touch the wound. I told him I needed a wee really badly. My voice came out as a whisper. Phil at first thought I was still circling the airport – how could I need a wee when I'd had nothing to drink since the day before? I repeated my need for the loo again and the Nurse brought a bedpan. I was mortified but felt too weak to get up and go to the toilet. Phil and the Nurse helped me on to it and I duly performed. It seemed only five minutes later when I needed another wee, and another wee after that. A stack of bedpans was hurriedly left in the room for my use. Fluids had been pumped through the cannula during the operation to keep me hydrated, and now they wanted to come out! I was piddling for England and also Ireland, Scotland and Wales for that matter. My little helper Phil became King of the Bedpans, and didn't flinch once in his duty.

My blood pressure, pulse and temperature were being closely monitored. The blood pressure and pulse were raised, but my temperature was normal. The Nurse was concerned about how fast my heart rate was. I could feel it pounding away in my chest even though I was lying still. The Doctor was called and came and duly did an ECG, but he said he wasn't concerned as the beat was regular. Whilst raising my gown to attach the ECG electrodes, a rash appeared on my chest which mysteriously vanished again in seconds. It seemed I was having some sort of reaction to the anaesthetic or pre-med or both. In my befuddled state, I hoped I wasn't going to have a heart attack. The Doctor went away and observations continued to be taken at regular intervals by the nursing staff.

I came to the realisation that I felt terribly weak and seemed to have no voice or coughing mechanism to speak of. My heart was racing and I couldn't turn my head from side to side as the stitches pulled in my neck. Not being able to cough properly was worrying as there suddenly seemed lots of phlegm on my chest that I was unable to shift which seemed to be getting stuck in the back of my throat. I couldn't believe I had gone from being reasonably fit to being struck down in a hospital bed hardly able to move within the space of a few hours.

More was to come. The Surgeon appeared in my room after completing his afternoon operating list. He thought it best to tell me that he didn't like the look of the thyroid gland that he'd taken out. In his experience it had looked possibly cancerous, and he'd sent it away to the laboratory to be analysed. He had also taken out four lymph nodes in my neck which had been swollen, and these too would be tested for cancer. I couldn't believe what I was hearing. It was like a bad dream that I couldn't wake up from. The Radiologist had assured me the lump was just a cyst, the Endocrinologist had told me it was ok to leave it alone if it wasn't causing problems, and now I was being told that the lump was probably cancerous. The Radiologist hadn't even thought it was necessary to perform a needle biopsy of the lower left thyroid, which almost certainly would have detected the cancer present. I didn't doubt the Surgeon at all. He'd had enough experience to know a cancerous thyroid when he saw one. I should have had surgery after the first ultrasound scan I thought – how much could the cancer have spread in the intervening six months? The Surgeon did add that thyroid cancer was easily treatable and my chances of survival would be in the region of 95 per cent. I would need radioactive Iodine (RAI) at a later date to kill off any thyroid cells left in my body and therefore kill the cancer contained within them. Thyroid cells are particularly partial to Iodine – they need it to make the hormone Thyroxine. After making any remaining thyroid cells sensitive to RAI by coming off the Thyroxine tablets I would need to take and eating a low-Iodine diet, the cells would then gobble up the RAI and be destroyed even if the cancer had spread elsewhere in the body (as any spread would be made up of thyroid cells). It sounded simple. I asked him where thyroid cancer usually spread to, and his answer was the lungs.

When the Surgeon left, Phil and I looked at each other, dazed. I didn't know what to say to my husband of nearly 25 years. I felt angry and sad at the same time. I did not want anybody feeling sorry for me, and I imagined Phil now being stuck with an invalid unable to work and a drain on the family finances. Phil being typically male did not show any reaction at all, looked on the bright side, and mentioned again the high survival rate and how it could be cured with the RAI. I knew though that he was trying to be cheerful and not show me how devastated he was. We couldn't believe this was happening. It was everyone's worst nightmare come true.

I lay back on the pillows and tried to sleep but the anaesthetic's after-effects ensured I would be wide awake for the next three days. When I did eventually doze off I woke up immediately feeling sick and dizzy each time, and this effect lasted for nearly two weeks after surgery. The amount of phlegm on my chest was bothering me, as I felt I was choking trying to cough it up. When the Hostess arrived with the supper for that first evening which I had ordered earlier in the day, I could not eat. I sipped water for the first day and night

CHAPTER EIGHT - SECOND DAY AFTER SURGERY

On the second day, a Nurse suggested I try and get out of bed to go to the toilet. This seemed like a monumental undertaking, as I felt so weak. I couldn't ever envisage being able to get in and out of the bath again either. The Nurse said not to try for a few days yet. Phil was on hand to help as I duly swivelled my legs around out of the bed and shakily stood up. My heart immediately started pounding again with the effort. I shuffled the few yards to the toilet and whilst in there made the mistake of looking at myself in the mirror.

My face was a strange brown rusty colour, which I attributed to an allergic reaction to the anaesthetic. The right side of my bottom lip was swollen and sore – goodness knows what had happened to that. An angry looking bright red scar about 3 inches long was present at the bottom of my neck, and below that was a big black bruise on my chest the size of a dinner plate. Horrified, I turned away and after going to the loo got thankfully back into bed. I would not win any beauty contests that day!

The Hostess arrived with my porridge and this time I could manage a few mouthfuls with a glass of fruit juice. Things were looking up - I still didn't feel sick and I had managed to jettison the bedpans. I was determined to walk to the toilet from now on. I even managed to have a little wash at the sink later in the day.

After breakfast was medicine time. The Nurse brought me a fast-acting Thyroxine substitute, Liothyronine Sodium (sometimes known as T3). I was to take three tablets per day. The tablets were 20micrograms each, and I would stay on these until two weeks before my RAI treatment when I would need to be off the T3 altogether and on a low Iodine diet. As mentioned before this was the only way to make any remaining thyroid cells hungry for Iodine and so receptive to the RAI, which would kill them off. If I had been on the proper LevoThyroxine hormone (sometimes known as T4), I would have had to come off it for six weeks prior to RAI treatment and would have felt very ill indeed (the T4 levels tend to stay constant in the body for longer, whereas T3 is short-acting and only takes two weeks to leave the body). That was the reason I was not given T4 LevoThyroxine immediately after surgery, as it took about six weeks to leave the body. It only takes about three months without Thyroxine for a person to die, so you can imagine how ill you would be after six weeks with no Thyroxine at all. It started to sound very complicated and I didn't feel much like trying to get my head around it at that moment. It was to take at least two weeks for the results of the biopsies to come back so I decided I'd worry about it then. It still might not be cancer. I was ever hopeful.

After medicine time and observations came the ward round. The Surgeon said I needed to stay another night but could go home the following day. Phil agreed that I would be better off at home, if nothing else it would improve my chances of sleep. I didn't feel well enough to go home actually, but went along with everybody else and welcomed the chance to leave hospital – it meant I was well and truly on the road to recovery.

Phil stayed with me for the rest of the day. I tried to doze but sleep eluded me. I was finding it hard to talk. I became out of breath if I tried to say too much all at once. Phil reassured me that because I could only whisper, I had to use more air for talking, which was causing the breathing problem. I was still having trouble coughing, and drinking anything made me splutter and choke. To cap it all I was also getting symptoms of yet another period coming. I couldn't believe it – one had only finished the week before after 19 days. Exactly the same thing was happening again which had caused me to consult a Gynaecologist ten years previously. I would have to go back on the Norethisterone tablets. Coupled with the new T4 LevoThyroxine tablets I would also have to take, I would be rattling. The improved diet was not good enough – I obviously had some major hormone deficiencies!

During the night I got out of bed to go to the toilet but felt very strange as I was walking back to bed. Pins and needles were in my hands and feet and I felt strangely light-headed. It wouldn't go away and I pressed the call button to summon the Nurse. She laid me down on the bed, raised my feet a little, and explained I'd had a little 'faint'. She checked my blood pressure, which was quite low. I'd never fainted before so didn't recognise the symptoms. She said I'd probably got out of bed too quickly, and was to sit on the bed for a few minutes first before getting out next time. I felt like an old lady. I could usually leap out of bed like a scalded cat.

The next day came and I was to go home after lunch. There would be a follow-up appointment two weeks later with the Surgeon in his clinic to hear the results of the biopsy. Phil brought the car as near to the back patio doors as he could as I was too weak to walk very far. I still didn't feel ready to go home, but said goodbye and thanks to the Nurses and Doctors, and held Phil's arm as he led me to the car. I sunk into the seat with a grateful sigh – the few yards had seemed like a long trek. We returned home via the GP's surgery. Phil dropped my discharge letter in and collected some more T3 Liothyronine Sodium tablets to see me through to the RAI treatment a couple of months down the line.

CHAPTER NINE – HOME AGAIN

When I arrived home on the Wednesday, it was early afternoon and Matt was not yet home from work. I couldn't be bothered to unpack my case and just sat on the sofa figuring out how to tell my son that I probably had cancer. There were also Lee and Sarah to tell who were coming to visit that evening and last but not least my eighty one year old mother who lived nearby. I quickly decided not to tell her, as she was a very anxious person who would doubtless have become very worried at the mention of the word 'cancer', and I couldn't have handled the dramatics in my delicate state. She would have possibly wrongly assumed I was dying and would have found it hard to listen to any explanation I would have been able to give. I would tell her my thyroid was removed along with a cyst in order to stop any more cysts growing on it. The Surgeon had assured me the survival rate was in the ninety to ninety-five per cent range, so I had high hopes that I wouldn't suddenly deteriorate and shuffle off.

I still felt rather dreadful. I had terrible trouble coughing up the large amount of phlegm that kept accumulating in the back of my throat. My cheeks had lost the rusty brown colour and now had a ghostly grey hue. I was still weak and could not walk far. When Matt was due home, I decided to soften the blow by putting a chiffon scarf around my neck so he could not see the damage done.

Matt bounded in his usual upbeat self and gave me a big hug. I relayed to him the Surgeon's probable diagnosis. His face fell, but he also said (as did Phil) that the survival rates were encouraging and of course there might not be any cancer found after the biopsy. He disappeared upstairs to bathe and change and seemed quiet after my revelation, only appearing for dinner and then returning to his room again where quiet acoustic guitar playing could be heard. Matt usually plays loud Rock and Melodic Metal, so something was wrong in his little world. Lee and Sarah popped over for a visit and the same scenario was played out. The look on their faces said it all. Lee went upstairs to talk to Matt for a while.

After Lee and Sarah's short visit, I had another coughing fit and thought I wouldn't be able to breathe suddenly with the amount of phlegm seemingly in the airway. I told Phil I needed to return to the Nuffield as I didn't feel safe at home with no emergency suction and felt I might drown in my own secretions. Fortunately my bag was still not unpacked. We told Matt I needed to go back to hospital. By this time it was 9.30 in the evening. Poor Phil felt dreadful as he blamed himself for encouraging me to come home believing it would be in my best interests. He phoned the Nuffield to tell them to expect us back and drove me there all stressed out and upset. I tried not to cough in the car in case I couldn't breathe in. I hoped no police were around hiding in lay-bys with hand-held mobile speed cameras as we raced back to the Nuffield in record time.

At 10pm we were ringing the night bell. It seemed an eternity before it was answered, as the Nurses on duty had been busy tending to patients and could not come down to open the door straight away. I was shown to a different room this time – room 23, which was not as nice as the one I had vacated that afternoon. It was upstairs with obviously no patio doors and garden. As soon as I arrived, I was seen by the admitting Nurse who took the usual pulse, temperature, and blood pressure, and then by the in-house Doctor who prescribed a course of nebulisers for me to inhale – 4 per day starting that night, to loosen the phlegm. Phil waited until I was settled inhaling the saline nebuliser (the machine was very loud and I'm certain kept the other patients nearby awake) and then went home to bed. I stayed connected to the nebuliser for half an hour or so, and it seemed to help. It was reassuring to be back in the hospital whilst I felt so unwell.

CHAPTER TEN – THREE DAYS AFTER SURGERY AND BEYOND

The next day was three days on from the surgery and I had a visit from the Physiotherapist who showed me some breathing exercises to do every half an hour that would give additional help with the phlegm problem. If I had known at the time it would take me about eight weeks to be almost rid of it I would have felt quite depressed! I must have had quite a bad reaction to the anaesthetic, as the phlegm certainly wasn't there before the operation. On a happier note I could not help but notice that the Physiotherapist was a tad on the hunky side (a girl can look can't she?), so I eagerly looked forward to learning further breathing exercises.

There was also a chest x-ray to be done. The Surgeon had requested this and Phil and I supposed he wanted to check for any secondary cancers. I was too weak to walk to the X-Ray Department, so a Porter came for me pushing a wheelchair. It took all my strength to stand up in front of the x-ray machine. Phil heard the Radiographer say to her colleague that she couldn't see any secondaries, which was encouraging. They told me the x-ray was clear. At least that was one piece of good news. The Surgeon also told me on the ward round my chest was clear and that if I felt better the next day, I could go home. The nebulisers were helping to loosen the phlegm, and I felt more able to cope. I agreed to go home the next afternoon.

On the Friday after lunch, we again said our goodbyes. It was a longer walk out of the hospital this time as we had to walk downstairs and then through the reception area and out to the car. I had my little chiffon scarf on again so as not to frighten any unsuspecting out-patients that were waiting in Reception. I chose to walk down the stairs rather than take the lift to prove to myself I could do it. I am terribly stubborn. It took an eternity but I did it clutching onto Phil's arm. I still looked and felt dreadful but somehow knew I wouldn't need to go back yet again.

Back at home I spent the next few weeks recuperating. I still could not move my neck from side to side properly, and to add to my troubles on the second day home, part of the cracked tooth broke off whilst I was eating dinner. Perhaps it had been knocked during the anaesthetising process. I felt like crying into my vegetables – how unlucky can one person get I thought? I felt too weak to manage a visit to the Dentist and decided to wait until I felt a bit better. Also during these first weeks my periods returned with such a vengeance that I was getting one every other week and constant PMT symptoms. I gave in and started taking the Norethisterone tablets again. At least one problem was solved. Another problem manifested itself though in the vacated space. I suspected the T3 dose of three tablets per day was too high as my heart was constantly pounding, I felt anxious, and was losing weight. I emailed the Surgeon who advised me to take two tablets instead, one in the morning and one in the evening, which seemed to agree with me more.

Luckily the weather was warm and I sat in the garden every day not doing much at all. At first Phil had to wash my hair and my back at bathtime as the movement pulled on the scar if I tried to do it, but after a couple of weeks I could do this for myself. I trawled the internet and joined a website run by other thyroid cancer sufferers. They had all gone through what I was experiencing and I found the site immensely helpful (www.thyroidcancersupportuk.org). I found thyroid cancer affects mainly middle-aged women and the cause was not known. There are theories that include too much weight gain and sudden weight loss during pregnancy, and radiation to the face or neck during childhood. Even Chernobyl was mentioned. I had had lots of dental x-rays as a child and teenager – perhaps that was the cause? I even toyed with the idea that the Norethisterone tablets that I had been taking for 10 years may have caused it, but could not find any evidence to support this. I still couldn't believe that this had happened to me as I had always taken care of my body. Even now in my weakened state I had started to walk around the village to regain my strength, usually taking the route I used to jog. I love to be outside, and as long as I could still walk, then as far as I was concerned I was ok.

On the 5th July, I attended the Nuffield as an out-patient to see the Surgeon and get the results of the biopsy. He confirmed I had Papillary thyroid cancer with spread to the surrounding lymph nodes (Stage T4 N1, so quite advanced), as the four swollen lymph nodes that had been removed were also cancerous. He explained Papillary cancer was the most common type and easily treatable (the other three types were follicular, medullary, and anaplastic thyroid cancer, with the latter two more difficult to treat successfully). I would have to undergo Radioactive Iodine (RAI) treatment at Addenbrooke's hospital to kill any remaining thyroid cells (and therefore any cancerous cells), and for this to happen he was going to refer me to a Consultant Oncologist who worked both at Addenbrooke's and at The Nuffield hospital in Cambridge. Yet another Doctor. He was also going to refer me to an Ear, Nose, and Throat (ENT) Consultant, to see if he could help with my lack of a voice. It still hadn't returned a couple of weeks after surgery and he was getting worried. If he was worried I was worried, and I wondered if it would ever come back. It was frustrating to try and talk and no voice came out and people could not hear me. Phil became my voice. I whispered into his ear and he translated to people who couldn't understand what I was saying. Over the next few weeks I regained five notes of the scale in the lower register but that was all. There was no power in the voice – if I was talking with one person in a room that was ok – I sounded like an adolescent schoolboy whose voice was breaking. But if I had to talk over background noise and tried to speak louder, nothing came out at all. I actually had to wait until December 2005 to see any real difference in my voice. By then, my speaking voice sounded normal, I had a range of 13 notes, but I still could not shout to get over any background noise (I still can't three years later).

On the 6th July I felt well enough to undergo repairs to the cracked tooth. Phil drove me to our Dentist in Long Melford who gave me a nice white filling. I think he must have felt sorry for me as he charged me the same price as the normal amalgam.

In the second week of July, about a month after the operation I attended Kidbrooke Comprehensive School's reunion of 'old girls'.

Looking back, I should have stayed at home as my voice was so weak and the background noise so loud that I could not make myself heard at all. My legs ached from following my friends around all the school corridors where I had run and skipped some thirty years before. With hindsight I realised the T3 levels were falling in the afternoon when I was doing lots of walking around the school (T4 does not cause the same symptoms as levels stay constant in the blood), and I was exhausted when Phil came to collect me in the car and slept most of the way home. The following day we were scheduled for a week away in the Isle of Wight (renting the bungalow again from Dave's sister) - this time just the two of us. Matt and Anna were off for a week's holiday in Italy, and Lee and Sarah stayed near the hospital as their baby was due the following week. It was a lovely week away from hospitals and Doctors. Just before we left for the Isle of Wight a letter arrived from the Oncologist with an appointment date to see her at the Nuffield hospital at Cambridge, which I noticed was the very next day after we were due home. I resolved to enjoy my holiday – the first holiday Phil and I had taken alone in over 23 years. We had always taken the boys with us on holiday and now they were grown up we finally had some time to ourselves. We could visit all those National Trust houses instead of children's playgrounds and arcades!

The weather was glorious as we left for the ferry and the sun didn't stop shining all week. We lazed on the beach at Puckpool, visited Osborne House and Arreton Manor, sunbathed in the secluded garden of the bungalow, and had a lovely dinner out every night near to the bungalow at The Windmill Hotel in Bembridge. Mary and Dave had been there the previous week and we met up on our first day for lunch before they went home. Only one cloud marred the horizon – the Thursday afternoon of that week saw me sitting in the Accident and Emergency department of the Isle of Wight's main hospital at Newport. My scar was sore and two places were infected and oozing pus. I wasn't sure what to do with it but the Doctor there said it was best to do nothing and leave it alone. He said the two infected places were caused by internal sutures sticking out of the scar. Eventually the stitches would drop out but it might take some time. When I got back to the bungalow I wiped the scar with salt water, which helped with the oozing but it still felt a bit sore.

There was a lovely end to the holiday on the Sunday morning when Lee phoned to tell us we were grandparents. Little Sophie Emily had been born by emergency caesarean the previous evening on July 16th 2005, and both mother and baby were doing well. We couldn't wait to catch the ferry back to see her. Although we weren't due to get on the ferry until midday, we caught the 9.30am ferry and by 2.30 pm were sitting outside the maternity ward waiting to see our new granddaughter, who of course was absolutely gorgeous.

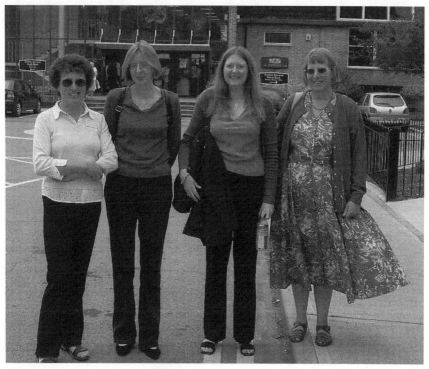

Myself (left) with some old schoolfriends at Kidbrooke School reunion, July 2005.

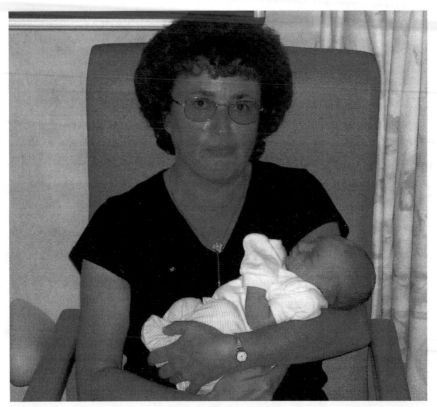

My little granddaughter Sophie at one day old July 17th 2005. Note the scar on my neck from the recent thyroidectomy one month earlier.

CHAPTER ELEVEN – THE FIRST RADIOACTIVE IODINE TREATMENT

Back to earth with a bump the next day back from holiday. Phil drove me to the Nuffield at Cambridge to meet a new Doctor on my ever-growing Doctors' Christmas card list. This time I would see a Consultant Oncologist. She felt my neck and asked how much I had been told of my condition. I filled her in with everything the Surgeon had told me and she nodded in agreement. She said she'd book me into the RadioIodine Suite at Addenbrooke's as soon as possible and I would have to come off my T3 (Liothyronine) tablets for two weeks beforehand in order for the RAI treatment to be effective. This I did not fancy much as I knew I'd feel weak and tired, but it had to be done. I would also have to be on a low Iodine diet to make any remaining thyroid cells hungry for the Iodine, so no fish or dairy products, and no food with red colouring in it. I didn't eat dairy anyway due to migraines, but it would be hard giving up fish. I would also have to wait for the keyhole surgery to repair my jaw, as she wanted the RAI treatment over with first. That meant taking even more time off work I thought, as now instead of September which I had planned, I would have to wait until probably the summer of 2006 for the locking jaw to be re-aligned. The Oncologist asked me if I wanted to stay a private patient or go through the NHS as the treatment was the same (apart from being treated sooner privately). I wanted it over with soon so told her I would remain a private patient. She said she would phone with the date of the RAI treatment later that day, and she gave me a compliment slip with all her contact numbers on and email address just in case I thought of any questions I wanted to ask her. I did indeed think of many questions over the next fortnight, and she always answered my emails. What a nice lady.

True to her word, she phoned that evening to give me the date of August 8th to go to Addenbrooke's for the start of the treatment. I would have to come off my T3 tablets the following Monday on 25th July. I immediately phoned our local restaurant/pub and booked a table for Sunday lunch – the last day when I could eat normally for a while. Lee and Sarah agreed to come to the lunch and bring baby Sophie along in her pushchair. I didn't know how long it would take to start feeling unwell, so I wanted to make the most of it. Dear little Sophie didn't murmur throughout the meal at all and we all enjoyed the afternoon.

In fact during the first week off the T3, I didn't feel too bad at all. I could still cut the grass on the Tuesday and take my mother shopping to Sainsbury's on the Friday. This is a doddle I thought. However the second week was quite different. I started feeling quite weary by the second Monday and was unable to do much at all. I had pains in my calf muscles when I tried to walk (muscles cannot contract properly without Thyroxine), and so developed a shuffling gait. I laid about on the sofa and wished it was all over. My eyes felt as though they had lead weights on the lids trying to hold them down. Phil had to help with the shopping on the second Friday as my legs refused to move much at all. I slept quite a bit during the day and because my sleep pattern was disrupted, had trouble sleeping properly at night. I looked and felt terrible. By the end of the fortnight my face was pale and puffy and I had put on half a stone in weight despite having a decreased appetite.

On the 8th August I dragged my poor suffering body through the revolving door of Addenbrooke's hospital. The admission letter had said arrive at the RAI Suite on Ward A5 at 10am. Due to my overeagerness to get there and start on the treatment we arrived an hour early. Because of the painful calf muscles I wanted to keep walking to a minimum, so I waited in the café by the entrance whilst Phil set about locating the ward. He returned after about 10 minutes having found it and spoken to one of the Nurses there who informed him we were too early and to come back at 10am! We stayed in the café reading the newspaper.

At 10am we went to the ward and were shown to the purpose-built RadioIodine Suite. At first I was a little disappointed as my room was quite small (one of two leading from a small lobby), and I would be holed up there all week. But at least it had windows which I could look out of (I thought it would be a lead-lined cell!), although there wasn't much of a view. The room also had a free telephone, a television, and my own sink and toilet. The shower room was just outside the door in the lobby. There was a kettle to make myself a hot drink and a toaster. Good thing I had brought some herbal tea bags I thought.

A Doctor came to take a blood test to check my haemoglobin, thyroglobulin (all thyroid cells produce thyroglobulin, so a high thyroglobulin level above 2 gives an indication that thyroid or thyroid cancer cells are still present), and TSH (thyroid stimulating hormone – which would be high as it had not been suppressed with T3 for a fortnight) levels. He explained that I would be given an anti-sickness pill about half an hour before the RAI drink. This would ensure it stayed down for the two or three hours it would take for my body to absorb it. After that I would need to be isolated and drink a lot of water and take frequent showers to flush it out of my system. He also tidied up the sutures which were still sticking out of the scar. A Nurse came in with admission paperwork which I helped her to fill in, and afterwards she gave me an identity wristband to wear. I asked when I could begin to take my T3 tablets again, and was told probably after my scan on Friday. Three weeks off T3 is no joke. The Physicist who would administer the drink arrived who checked my identity and more or less repeated what the Doctor said. I couldn't go home unless radioactive levels were safe for me to be let out into the community. When he left I looked at Phil and sighed. At last things were underway. I was due to fight my own little war alone in this room against an unseen enemy.

I was then visited by Ann who had worked on the RAI Unit for 16 years. Ever cheerful, it was her job to bring me my meals. She explained that when I was radioactive, she would knock at the door and if I left my table near to the door and sat as far away from the door as possible, she would leave my meals on the table. I would then wash up my plate and cutlery and leave them outside the room for her to collect at a later date when all the rooms had been decontaminated. She brought me a nice lamb stew at midday and some extra pillows and towels. She even said if I gave her the correct change before my RAI drink, she would buy a newspaper for me every day. What a star! If I had left the ward highly radioactive to go down to the shop, I would have set off a loud alarm bell just outside the RAI suite!

After lunch, Phil and I sat about and waited for the RAI drink. At 1.30 I was given an anti-emetic and at 3pm the Physicist returned with the drink, which was Phil's cue to leave. He wouldn't be able to visit again until the next day when radioactive levels had dropped somewhat, and then only for 20 minutes each day. He had to enter the room wearing plastic overshoes and gloves and sit as far away from me as possible.

The Physicist had a rather large bottle in his hand and my face fell at the thought of having to drink the whole contents – no wonder they gave the anti-emetic first! He laughed and said no, the bottle contained a liquid that I was to sprinkle down the toilet before flushing it which would help to break up the RAI. The drink itself came in a lead-lined box and was only a tiny amount. He checked my identity again with the Nurse present, and then inserted 2 needles into the top of the RAI phial. These were attached to 2 plastic tubes, one of which I would drink through like a straw. The end of the other one he put into a cup of water which helped to flush the last of the RAI out of the phial and into me, ensuring I had all of it.

I duly drank the RAI after putting on a plastic apron to guard against splashes, and that was that. The Physicist left after taking the first readings. Apparently levels would need to be one quarter of the present reading before I could go home. I resolved to wait half an hour to let the RAI go down before I started drinking. After that, I drank as much water as I felt able to for the rest of the day. Tea consisted of soup and sandwiches, which were put outside my door at 5pm after a call from the reception desk asking if I wanted them. I spent the evening reading, filling in crossword puzzles, and watching television. I made use of the free phone to call Phil, Matthew, and my mother.

The night passed uneventfully as far as feeling nauseous was concerned. I tossed and turned though as air-conditioning units outside droned constantly and the fridge hummed and buzzed inside. At 7am I phoned the desk to make sure I had enough time to take a shower before breakfast. Staff seemed quite helpful and I was assured Ann would leave my breakfast until last, giving me enough time to wash. After that it was time to occupy myself until the Oncologist did her ward round and the Physicist returned to check if my radiation levels had decreased.

After lunch consisting of sausages, mash, and vegetables, the Oncologist popped her head round the door. She said as soon as the Physicist said radiation levels were ok, I could go home and then come back Friday for a body scan. I could start back taking my T3 tablets the next day, Wednesday. Awesome! I couldn't wait to be able to walk properly and feel normal again instead of exhausted all the time. I had found out through the internet support group, that there were Thyrogen injections I could have had to stimulate my TSH levels without coming off the T3 tablets. The Oncologist's colleague had said the NHS wouldn't fund the injections as they were £250 each, but my medical insurance company would probably pay for them. I made a mental note to ask the Oncologist about them during my next follow-up appointment with her at the Nuffield, Cambridge, on September 12th to get my blood test findings and scan results. I would also probably need a second increased dose of RAI in six months time to ensure all cancer cells had been killed off.

On that second day, the Nurses kept asking if I needed anti-sickness pills as though they were all waiting for me to throw up. I felt I was disappointing them munching my way through all meals put in front of me!

The Physicist arrived about 2.30 to check radiation levels. He nodded encouragingly and said levels were a third below the previous day's readings and all being well I could go home the next day. I nearly jumped for joy as it was only a small room and I was getting a touch of cabin fever. I much prefer being outside, so it had been hell.

Phil arrived at 6.15pm for his allotted 20 minutes. He wanted to stay longer but wasn't allowed. The poor chap was sweating in his rubber gloves and plastic overshoes.

As soon as I woke up on the Wednesday, down the little red lane went the first T3 tablet for nearly 3 weeks. I had to take T3's for one week, and then the proper T4 Levothyroxine tablets from then on which would keep my TSH suppressed and hopefully stop any more thyroid/thyroid cancer cells from growing. I noticed my salivary glands were starting to feel a little sore and my mouth was dry so I sucked on some boiled sweets which I had been advised to bring, as they would help by stimulating the salivary glands. The trouble was I wasn't too keen on boiled sweets, and so could only manage a couple. Lunch was a nice chicken and leek pie with vegetables and then mixed fruit afterwards.

The Oncologist visited as usual at 2pm and confirmed I could eat normally when I returned home – no more low Iodine diet. I also wouldn't need a certificate of radiation given when we embarked on our cruise in November. I was worried I might have set off airport alarms but she felt sure this wouldn't happen.

At 2.30 the Physicist made his usual rounds. He said radioactive levels were low enough for me to go home. He checked all my belongings and said only the clothes I had been wearing were slightly radioactive, but if I washed them separately when I got home and then run the washing machine again empty, that would solve the problem. I could not prepare any food that evening, I was to stay away from public places for the rest of the day, and pregnant women and children for another 3 days. After that I would be back to normal. I was to return for the scan on Friday and could collect my new 200mcg T4 Thyroxine tablets from the ward then which would see me through for the next month. I would then need to order them on a repeat prescription from the GP. Luckily I had also found out on the support group that by having a chronic long-term medical condition needing Levothyroxine tablets, I would be exempt from prescription charges for life. There is an advantage to having thyroid cancer! Phil arrived at 5.30 to take me home. It was lovely walking out into the fresh air. I'd only had to stay in for 3 days so all in all the first RAI dose hadn't been as bad as I'd first thought.

CHAPTER TWELVE – RESULT OF TREATMENT AND 1ST GAMMA SCAN

Funnily enough it was the next day at home when I felt at my worst. My salivary glands felt swollen and sore, I felt sick after dinner, and I still had aching legs and exhaustion from the lack of T3 tablets. I knew it would take quite a few days for the T3 to kick back in, but I sobbed as I wanted to feel better NOW!

On the Friday it was time to return to Addenbrooke's for a Gamma scan. Phil noticed I was walking better along the hospital corridors. Thinking about it, yes, my calf muscles weren't as painful. The T3 was starting to work at last. I was still tired, but there was a definite improvement from the day before.

At the Nuclear Medicine department before my scan, the Technician asked me to empty my bladder, drink a cup of water to wash any radioactivity from the salivary glands, and remove any metal objects before getting me to climb onto the scanner bed. There were large camera plates above and below me. The Technician told me the plates would come quite close to my face but wouldn't actually touch me, and would take pictures from my head to just below my pelvis. I felt rather apprehensive as I suffer from mild claustrophobia and my heart started racing. The Technician reassured me she would be in the room with me at all times. I decided to shut my eyes when the bed moved inside the camera plates so that I wouldn't feel shut-in, and try to project my mind away from it all. The plates seemed to stay close by my head for ages before I could see more light behind my eyes and sensed they had moved downwards. I opened my eyes and relaxed somewhat after that as my head was outside the scanner. The scan took about 30 minutes and I had to lie as still as possible. No results could be seen straight away. Unfortunately I would have to wait for one month.

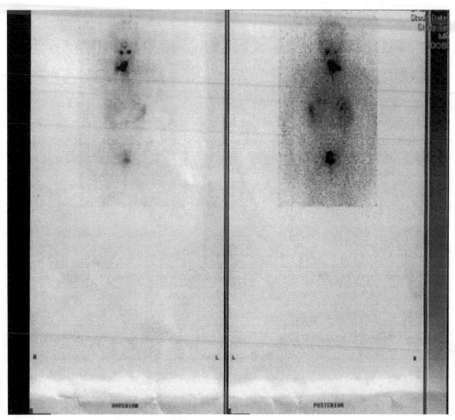

1ˢᵗ scan pictures taken on 12ᵗʰ August 2005 showing uptake of RAI in the thyroid bed. There is always uptake in the salivary glands and bladder, so these are discounted.

On the first Sunday after my treatment it was wonderful walking along Great Yarmouth seafront. Although the usual east wind was blowing and there was rain in the air, it was a positive tonic after being shut in earlier in the week in the little room on Ward A5. Phil and I sat and froze on the beach and loved every minute of it (well, I did anyway).

When the following Wednesday came around, I could start on the new T4 Levothyroxine tablets that I would have to take for the rest of my life. The nursing staff on Ward A5 had said to take them with food as they could be 'rough on the stomach'. The instructions on the packet and the internet support group for thyroid cancer sufferers said to take them first thing in the morning without food. My GP said it didn't matter one way or the other. I was totally unsure what to do and emailed the Oncologist. Back came the answer that it was best to take them on an empty stomach first thing in the morning.

The only drawback I can see from having cancer, is that if any other medical condition presents itself, one immediately thinks the cancer must be returning. Since May I had had a round spot in my vision in my right eye and a couple of weeks after my stay at Addenbrooke's, I was back at my local hospital's Eye Clinic as an NHS patient. I think I am destined never to go too long without a hospital visit. The appointment had been put off since just before my thyroidectomy, and as I sat waiting to see the Doctor, I wondered if the cancer had spread to my eye. I told myself not to be so stupid and to wait and see what the Doctor would say. I was told there was a leaky blood vessel on my retina which was causing the spot, it was nothing to do with the cancer – it was just one of those things that happen sometimes. It looked to be resolving itself though, but just to be on the safe side, I would have to come back in a few weeks' time and have an injection of an Iodine based dye so that the Medical Photographer could take some pictures and see if the blood vessel was still leaking. If it was, it could be zapped with a laser. I thought I'd better check with the Oncologist to see if this procedure (called a Fluorescein Angiography) would be ok for me to undergo, as I would be pumped with Iodine again.

I got to see her again at her monthly Thyroid Clinic at Addenbrooke's. Although I had an appointment to see her on 12th September at Cambridge's Nuffield hospital, another appointment had come through the post for 6th September for the NHS Thyroid Clinic at Addenbrooke's, which had probably been automatically generated by the staff on Ward A5. Phil and I duly made our way to the clinic on the 6th September. I was nervous, as I knew I would probably get the result of the scan and was worried that the cancer had spread. I imagined chemotherapy, losing my hair, having to cancel our 25th anniversary cruise booked for 18th November – my imagination was running riot and my heart was beating fast (catastrophising I think they call it!)

My heart sank when I saw the queue of people sitting in Clinic 12's waiting area on that Tuesday morning. Everybody had scars on their necks though, so I felt right at home. As Phil and I were looking round for a seat, the Oncologist walked past and asked what we were doing there as she hadn't expected to see me until the following Monday at the Nuffield. That was a good start.

Fortunately I was called right on time. I sat down in the consulting room next to Phil and thought my heart would burst out of my chest as it was pounding so much. I had nothing to fear. The Oncologist explained that the uptake of the Radioiodine had all been in my neck area only, so the cancer had not spread (as far as she could tell). I breathed a sigh of relief. I would need another dose of RAI the week beginning January 16th 2006 as my thyroglobulin level was above normal and the scan showed uptake in the neck area, but in the meantime could go on my cruise, have holiday vaccinations, and have my Iodine dye injected in my local hospital's Eye Clinic. Also I was told to forget about Doctors and hospitals until January! I just needed a blood test so that she could check if I had enough Thyroxine in my system to keep the thyroid stimulating hormone suppressed. I was also told I could have Thyrogen injections before my second RAI treatment, so that I wouldn't need to come off the T4 tablets (apparently with the first RAI dose it is advisable to always come off the T3 tablets and have Thyrogen injections on subsequent treatments). I nearly floated out of the consulting room and didn't even mind the long wait in Addenbrooke's blood testing area. Phil seemed even more relieved than I was and we hurriedly posted off the outstanding balance for the cruise on the way home (I had kept the money back in case we had to cancel due to my ill-health, chemotherapy etc.). At Addenbrooke's I had seen a fellow sufferer from the internet support group who was also waiting for a blood test. She had undergone not only a thyroidectomy, but two neck dissections as well due to spread to the lymph nodes. Her neck looked like a map of the Norfolk broads. I thanked my lucky stars I only had one small scar.

The week following the visit to the Thyroid Clinic was nearly six weeks after my first dose of Radioactive Iodine. It had taken all this time for the T4 Levothyroxine levels to come up, and I was noticing that my heart was pounding at a very fast rate even when I was sitting still, and that my body was giving off so much heat that my glasses were steaming up on the inside! I had a nasty feeling the dose was too high so I emailed the Oncologist and waited for her reply. She emailed back saying the results of the blood test at the Thyroid Clinic showed that the Thyroxine dose of 200mcg was too high and that I was to reduce to 175mcg per day. That was fair enough, but I only had 100mcg tablets. Yet another visit to the GP surgery ensued to get some 50mcg and 25mcg tablets, as the 100mcg tablets were too small to cut up accurately. Now I would have to wait for another six weeks for the new dose to stabilise and then have another blood test to check the level. Having thyroid cancer treatment seemed a very long-drawn out process I was beginning to realise!

On the 21st September I faced yet another doctor but this time back at the Nuffield at Bury St Edmunds. This time it was the Consultant ENT Surgeon and I was hoping there would be something he could do for my weak voice. I still only had a few tones in the lower register after three months and a kind of two-tone breathy whisper in the upper regions. Singing was out of the question, which was making me quite depressed, as I am a very musical person and to sing along to a song was second nature to me. The ENT Surgeon gave me a local anaesthetic through my nose which numbed the back of my throat (fortunately) and he then began threading a camera on the end of a long tube through my nose down the back of my throat so that he could see the vocal cords. The experience was most disagreeable, and I had to use the 'shut my eyes and project my mind away from it all' strategy. He asked me to count to ten. He could see as I was talking that my left vocal cord was paralysed and that the right one was trying to compensate, but to not much effect. The nerve had either been severed or damaged through manipulation during the operation. The Endocrine Surgeon had told him he had had trouble in removing my lymph glands, so the manipulation had probably caused the damage. The ENT Surgeon suggested leaving well alone for at least six months to see if the vocal cord improved, as in his experience there was often improvement six to nine months later, and he didn't want to operate and then find afterwards the vocal cord had healed by itself, thus

CHAPTER THIRTEEN – NEW JOB & VISIT TO THE EYE CLINIC

Meanwhile my workplace managers were starting to wonder when I would be returning to work. My Ward Manager had envisioned I would need only three weeks off work initially to recover. This had stretched to nearly four months as although I felt recovered, my voice was so weak I knew I would not be able to answer the phone which rang constantly on the ward, or be able to do much talking to ward visitors. I had frittered away the whole summer sitting outside on my favourite piece of garden furniture, the 'Timewaster' (a kind of swinging chair with a canopy). The Clinical Manager suggested a meeting on September 22nd which I duly attended. After I had told her my problems with speaking for any length of time, she suggested re-deployment and asked me if I would be interested in a Secretarial Assistant vacancy in the Cardiology Department, as she had had only good reports regarding my work and she wanted to give me a chance to work again. The job would mostly involve typing letters and reports. I couldn't believe my luck. Not only was a Secretarial Assistant a grade 3 post (my current post was grade 2) so there would be a higher salary, it was the sort of job I had been after for some time but somebody else always beat me to it. This time I would face no competition – the job was mine! I was to start work on 3rd October. I positively skipped back to the car – I had begun to think that due to my illness I would be on the scrapheap regarding work and job prospects. How wrong I was! I would be on a three months trial and I vowed to work as hard as I could to show them how well I could do the job. There would be times when I would have to take time off to have treatment in the Eye Clinic and to undergo Radioactive Iodine therapy at Addenbrooke's, so I hoped that people didn't feel sorry for me and think I was totally unhealthy and a lost cause.

I spent the next week excitedly shopping for new work clothes and spending a great deal of my September's salary in the process. October 3rd arrived, and feeling very nervous I reported as asked to the Manager who was in charge of all the Secretaries. She took me along to my new office upstairs situated in the corridor of the new Cardiology ward. There were two Secretaries there who turned out to be very friendly, helpful, and went out of their way to answer any questions I had, and I had many. There was a whole new specialised vocabulary to learn, names of drugs to learn how to type and audio typing to get to grips with, especially deciphering the heavily accented voices coming at me through the headphones. Within a week I knew I loved the job and wanted to stay there. The other girls helped me as much as they could during that first week including the other two part-time Secretaries who only worked a couple of days a week each.

I thought I would feel really tired that first week, but as I was sitting down for most of the day I did not feel too bad – I had felt more tired in my previous job at the end of the day in which I had been much more active. I was beginning to get back to my normal self, the only nagging pains were an occasional pain in my left collar bone and the teeth on the right side of my mouth were sometimes painful but I had a high pain threshold and decided to live with it. The hardest thing of all was trying to reassure myself that not every pain was the cancer coming back – it was probably the aches and pains of getting older. I was still feeling hot most of the time though, and suspected the 175mcg Thyroxine was still too high. Blood tests revealed this was so, and I was switched to 150mcg and felt a good deal better on this dose, but still hot sometimes. However I was still over-medicated but the Oncologist did not want me to come down any more, as 150mcg was keeping the TSH level suppressed which would hopefully stop any more thyroid cancer tissue from growing, and she thought it dangerous to drop the dose to 125mcg as that was too low. I would have to be over-medicated for the rest of my life. I read that too much Thyroxine in the system made you susceptible to osteoporosis, and resolved to ask the Oncologist about that when I went to Addenbrooke's in January for my second RAI dose.

October 3rd was also memorable for another reason. Having gone to bed happy at the way my first day back at work had gone, I was woken up by Matthew at 1.30am. He never usually wakes me up. I assumed he was sick but he assured me he was not. He then dropped a bombshell that kept me awake for the rest of the night worrying and fretting. He had found a lump in his testicle whilst showering that evening and the poor boy had been lying in bed obviously worried to death until he just had to tell somebody. I told him that he needed to be seen by the GP as soon as possible to get it investigated, and he agreed. I took pains to tell him just because he had a lump, it didn't mean he had cancer – it could be anything. He went back to bed but neither of us slept – I had only just finished Lance Armstrong's autobiography about how he beat testicular cancer and went on to win the Tour de France seven times, and what with my family's medical history, I must admit I feared the worst. However, a visit to the Doctor's surgery the next day reassured all of us. The GP was almost 100% sure it was a twisted vas deferens and made an appointment for Matthew to have a scan to confirm it. My son's face after coming home from the Doctor's was a picture of happiness. I only hoped the Doctor knew what he was talking about, and that my diagnostic nightmare was not about to be repeated with Matt. We awaited the appointment for the scan. Only the week before I had said to Phil something along the lines of 'I wonder what else God is going to throw at us in 2005'. The appointment for the scan arrived and was scheduled for October 24th. Thankfully all was well and was just as the Doctor had diagnosed.

I had only been at my new job for 3 weeks when it was time to take another day off for my Fluorescein angiograph of my eye on October 20th. First of all the Nurses tested my vision by getting me to read the letter chart. This I managed with flying colours – so far so good. Then it was time to have some local anaesthetic drops put in my eyes and drops to dilate my pupils so that the Technician could take the photos of the back of my eye. A cannula was put in my hand for the dye to be injected into, and then I was taken into the photography room. The whole procedure was rather unpleasant as when the pupils are dilated you are very sensitive to bright lights. As the dye was injected into the cannula, the Technician snapped away, but each photo was accompanied by a brilliant flash of light that gave me a headache by the end of it. Being an allergic sort of girl, the Nurse was concerned that I might feel sick or faint as the dye was injected, but happy to

CHAPTER FOURTEEN – HAPPIER TIMES

Yet more time was to be taken off work from November 18th to December 5th, but this time for a much happier reason. Phil and I finally had the dream holiday that we'd promised ourselves years back when the boys were growing up and we'd spent countless holidays in children's playgrounds. We really pushed the boat out so to speak and went on a P&O cruise to the Caribbean on their newest cruise ship 'Arcadia'. It was really to celebrate our 25th wedding anniversary which had fallen on October 11[th,], but I suppose we were also celebrating my new lease of life. We had a wonderful time visiting Barbados, Grenada, Dominica, Tortola, Catalina Island, Grand Cayman, Costa Maya, Cozumel, and Fort Lauderdale in the good old USA. The ship was a massive floating paradise catering to our every whim, and the Goanese crew did everything they could to make our holiday special. The temperature averaged 82°F every day and Christmas seemed a long way away when you were sitting on a Caribbean beach (back home it was snowing with ho-ho-hoing Santas appearing in every shop window)! We flew home from Miami airport on 3rd December to temperatures somewhat lower!

Two other happy events presented themselves in December. I was told my three- month trial at work was up and I could keep my new job – it was on a fixed-term basis but my Manager had every faith that my contract would be renewed each year. She even said she was pushing for it to be a grade higher (more money!). Also I was aware that six months after the thyroidectomy, my voice had suddenly become much better. Up until the end of October I had only a five maybe six note range, but a month or so later I could sing one octave plus two more notes – 12 notes in all! The relief! I could sing along to all my CD's in my car on the way to work. I noticed I had to take more breaths than before when I tried to sing though, and could not manage to sing a fast song all the way through, as I would be gasping for breath. I could just about manage if it was a slow song though. Maybe the Consultant

ENT Surgeon would not need to repair my vocal cord after all? He had referred me to an NHS speech therapist and when I came back from holiday there was a letter telling me I was now on the waiting list. What with my body slowly repairing itself and speech therapy, maybe there would be one operation cancelled and only one more to go (the jaw)? I would still go along to my appointment with the ENT Surgeon in March, but was starting to think that maybe nothing would need to be done. It would be a good Christmas this year for me. Not so for poor old Rick Parfitt from one of my favourite Rock bands Status Quo, who had to cancel the rest of Quo's UK tour as a growth had been found on his larynx. He was due to have exploratory surgery the week before we were to attend a Quo concert on 17th December at Wembley. Poor old Rick would probably never sing again as they already suspected cancer. It had worked out all right so far for me, but I had my doubts about Rick. I had no need to worry. Rick was soon to be back rocking, as the nodes were benign. He could enjoy his Christmas with his family. His voice was never the same afterwards though, but good for him to not give up touring and singing with the band. He was going to Rock 'till he dropped. My sentiments exactly.

Christmas arrived with its usual flurry of visiting relatives and relatives to be visited. Christmas Day lunch was spent at the Punch and Judy pub in Cardinal Park, Ipswich, with Lee, Sarah, Sophie (good as gold all day – never murmured!) Matt, Anna, and my mother. Boxing Day was spent at Phil's parents' house in Hastings, and there was a New Year's Eve dance and buffet at the Riverside Club in Stowmarket with Matt, Anna, Anna's parents and a couple of their friends. It was the perfect Christmas that was spoilt by only one thing. Over the Christmas holidays I had found a dark round lump inside my mouth on my right inner cheek. I did not tell a soul all over Christmas, especially Phil, as I did not want to spoil anyone's fun. I did tell him when the holidays were over, but nobody else knew. His face gave away no indication as to his thoughts. I was hoping the lump might have gone away during the holidays, but it hadn't. I wondered hopefully if the lump was due to my sometimes accidentally biting the inside of my mouth due to my jaw being out of alignment. I often woke in pain due to biting my cheek inadvertently whilst asleep. Finally I knew what I had to do. At the beginning of January I emailed my Oncologist and she quickly replied that she had got me an appointment with a colleague of hers at the Maxillo-Facial clinic at Addenbrooke's on the morning of 16th January when I was due to go in anyway for my second dose of radioactive Iodine. Hey ho - another Doctor! I was beginning to fear I had another type of cancer. I had only just drawn a line under 2005 and now cancer was rearing its ugly head again. The thought that I might have the big C a second time dominated my thoughts during the early days of 2006.

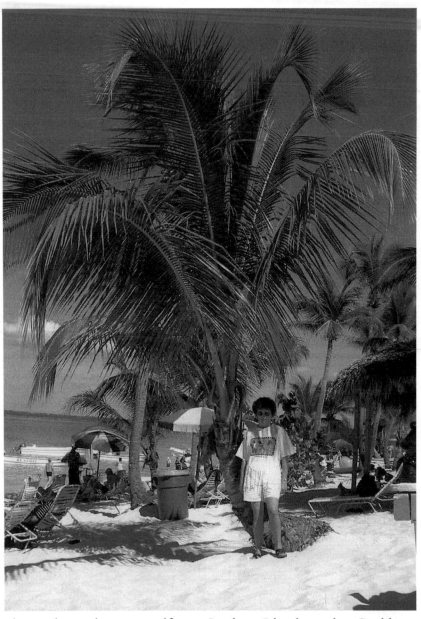

Photo above shows myself on Catalina Island in the Caribbean, November 2005.

CHAPTER FIFTEEN – SECOND RADIOACTIVE IODINE TREATMENT

Monday January 16th came round far too soon and Phil and I started off early for my week's stay in Addenbrooke's for the second radioactive Iodine dose and to attend the Maxillo-Facial Clinic. This time the District Nurse had visited me during the previous two days to administer two doses of Thyrogen (total cost £500 thankfully paid by medical insurance) by intramuscular injection. This at least spared me the listlessness, weight gain, pain on walking etc. that had dogged me the last time when I had to come off the T3 tablets. The Oncologist said it was necessary only for the first dose of radioactive Iodine to stop taking T3. Thankfully this time I had carried on as normal and gone to work. If I had had to stop taking my Thyroxine tablets I would not have been able to work after a few days and yet more time would have had to be taken off. The Thyrogen injections made any remaining thyroid cells receptive to the Radioactive Iodine. Coming off of Thyroxine would have done the same job also, but I would have felt tired as before and not be able to walk properly. Thankfully I suffered no ill-effects from the injections, despite the long list of side-effects contained in the blurb that came with the Thyrogen powder. After the first injection (embarrassing because the injection was in my behind and administered by a District Nurse who had worked on my ward when I was a Ward Clerk) I sat there and waited to throw up, faint, run to the loo, or goodness knows what else, but nothing happened at all.

We firstly visited the Maxillo-Facial Outpatients' Clinic where I was to be seen by the Addenbrooke's Oral Surgeon, but unfortunately the reception staff there knew nothing about me. Enquires were made to Ward A5 where I would once again be staying on the Iodine Suite, and surprisingly he was waiting for me there in my little room. Back we trooped to Ward A5 to be told by the Oral Surgeon that the lump was nothing to worry about, it was self-inflicted due to me biting the inside of my mouth whilst asleep. Well, that was a weight off my shoulders. It had been troubling me all over Christmas in case it had been a secondary.

The routine seemed unchanged from the first time I stayed on the ward. Cheery Ann was still there giving out meals. I was given the other room this time, so at least it was a change from the familiar four walls of the first room. The Physicist visited during the afternoon and administered a slightly higher dose of radioactive Iodine than before that would hopefully kill off any thyroid cells left. Then it was the usual drinking, showering and sitting about for a couple of days waiting to be told I was no longer emitting radiation and I could leave the room and go home. I was pleased to discover that I was suffering no side-effects this time. The Oncologist had told me that the second time around there is less thyroid tissue for the radiation to cling to (it doesn't cling to any other part of the body except the thyroid) and the radiation tends to leave the body quicker. The first time I experienced painful salivary glands, but on the second visit there was nothing.

The boredom was intense though, and the RadioIodine suite was so hot that I wanted to climb out of the window (it wouldn't open far enough) and feel the cold fresh air on my face (hyperthyroid patients are very intolerant to heat). Because it was winter, the heat was on full blast. I hate heat. The food was terrible – much worse than before. I could only think hospital finances must have been severely strained when only fatty mincemeat and dubious unrecognisable offerings came my way. Thank goodness for Phil bringing in fruit and fruit smoothies made by his own sausage fingers. The dear man had also bought me a portable DVD player for Christmas, so I was able to pass a few pleasant hours watching my favourite films.

I remembered to ask the Oncologist about osteoporosis when she visited my room (being over-medicated on Thyroxine can cause this). She said there was only a slight risk but she would organise a bone scan in the future, about two years down the line. Funnily enough, an uninvited letter from the Mobile Bone Density Screening Service had arrived in the post the week before, inviting me to pay £35 for a bone ultrasound scan for osteoporosis. My medical records were obviously easily available on computer, and they thought they'd target me I suppose as I was on too much Thyroxine. I thought it was a good idea though and made an appointment for Saturday January 21st.

I was allowed to go home, as before, on the Wednesday afternoon (I virtually ran out of the ward and down the stairs, eager to get outside) and was to come back for a scan two days later. The results of the scan and the blood tests taken (to determine thyroglobulin levels which gives an indication if any more thyroid cells are present) would not be available for another two months. I decided to forget about the results for the whole of the intervening time and not worry about it at all, as I would have been a nervous wreck by my appointment date at Cambridge's Nuffield Hospital on Monday March 13th. The scan was easier to tolerate as this time as I was allowed to play my 'Queen with Paul Rodgers' CD, so I kept my eyes shut and concentrated on the music, trying to forget the enormous camera plate was centimetres from my nose. The Technicians appreciated the music as they were heartily cheesed off with Addenbrooke's grim choices of Sixties' singalong CD's. I suppose many of the patients were teenagers back in the Sixties, but unfortunately the Technicians were not.

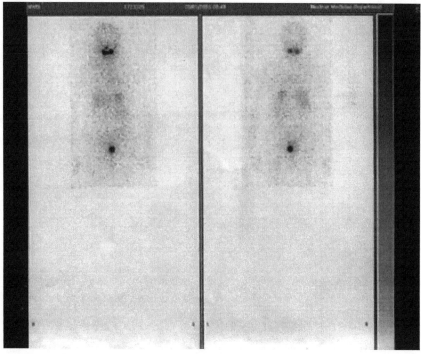

Scan on 20th Jan 06 showing RAI uptake in salivary glands and bladder only (usual).

Finally that was it. I could get back to normal and return to work the following Monday. The second dose had been given and hopefully I would be given the all clear in March and not need a third dose.

The following weekend I attended the Mobile Bone Density Screening Unit parked in a local GP surgery car park. All I had to do was take off the sock and shoe from my left foot (as I am right-handed I was told the left side was a little weaker) and place my foot upon the small scanner. The heel was always scanned, as it was the greatest weight-bearing bone. Some acoustic gel was placed on both sides of my foot near the heel, and the scanner then did its thing for a few minutes. The result was so good that the operator decided to do a scan on my right foot as well to check there wasn't a mistake. All that jogging over the previous 10 years had strengthened my bones and on the resultant graph where the central black reference line to aim for was 100%, I was 139%! Some good results for a change! Unfortunately although the jogging does give you strong bones, it does nothing for the joints and I was starting to get achy knees from time to time. I still felt good after a jog though, and had started it up again when my strength returned as I enjoyed it so much. At least I wasn't going to get osteoporosis in the near future. Unfortunately the jogging would end for good in the spring, as my knees started to become painful when I ran. I was still determined I would do some kind of exercise, and from then on began to walk as fast as I could for at least half an hour every day. The knees stopped hurting, and all was well.

CHAPTER SIXTEEN – ALL CLEAR?

I couldn't bear to be away from a hospital for too long, so I decided to bring forward my appointment to see the ENT Surgeon at Bury's Nuffield hospital. Since the beginning of February my nose had been sore and bleeding from time to time. Phil mentioned going to see the GP about it, but I thought it wasn't worth it as he would have only referred me to an ENT Consultant and I had been due to see him in March about my voice anyway. I phoned the Nuffield and brought my appointment forward to 15th February. I felt certain he would tell me my vocal cord was working again as I seemed to be speaking normally as long as there wasn't any loud background noise.

The ENT Surgeon placed the hated scope in my nostril and down the back of my throat (thankfully he gave me another local anaesthetic that numbed the gagging reflex). He again asked me to count from one to ten. Unfortunately he could see that the vocal cord was still paralysed, but the other one was compensating quite well. He said there was an operation he could do to strengthen it, but as my voice wasn't too bad I would not notice much of a difference. In my nose he could see a raw patch on the septum. He didn't think it was to do with my 'other business' (never heard of cancer of the nose!), but thought it was an infection for which he prescribed some antibiotic cream. I was to return in a month's time so he could look at my nose again. He didn't think it was worth doing anything regarding the voice until at least a year had passed since the operation, and it had only been eight months. Disappointed that my vocal cord was still paralysed and probably always would be, I left the consulting room and made another appointment for 15th March.

Over the next couple of weeks my nose started to feel better and was not so tender. The bleeding stopped and I did not think the ENT Surgeon would find anything when he looked a second time.

Meanwhile back at work things were moving on apace. I had only been in my new secretarial job since October when my Manager approached me mid-February to ask whether I would like a Grade 4 Medical Secretary's post, as I was coping well with Grade 3 work, my current post was only temporary, and she wanted me to be in a permanent post. Since becoming a Medical Secretary had been my original aim back in 2002 when I joined the NHS, I quickly said yes. I couldn't believe my luck at the way things were turning out. I only hoped I'd be up to the job which I knew could be very pressurised, with phones ringing constantly and a constant backlog of work to process. I was able to talk normally on the telephone now, so that was in my favour. I was to work for a world-renowned Pain Consultant, his Associate Specialist, a team of Clinical Nurse Specialists, an Acupuncturist, and a Pain Counsellor. I would be typing clinic letters, booking appointments for patients, sorting administration, and answering the telephone etc.

With much trepidation I started work as a Medical Secretary in the Pain Department on Wednesday February 22nd 2006. For the first few days most of it went straight over my head, but I slowly started getting to grips with it and found I was enjoying it and had found my little niche in life. The much-in-demand Pain Consultant had thriving private and NHS practices, and gave lectures all over the world on pain relief. It had taken thyroid cancer to get me the job I wanted in the first place! If I hadn't lost my voice I would probably still have been a Ward Clerk. The saying 'every cloud has a silver lining' was definitely true for me!

To top it all, the Oncologist emailed me at the beginning of March to say that my thyroglobulin (Tg) level had decreased from 4.9 at the first RAI dose down to 1.5 by the second, which was within normal limits (normal being 2 or less). Over time my Tg count would decrease even more to undetectable levels once the TSH was suppressed again. Also my 2nd scan had shown no abnormal uptake, so I could consider myself free from disease! The Oncologist still wanted to see me though on

13th March to show me the scan pictures and to inform me of future check-up procedures. The new year was definitely turning out better than the previous!

The Oncologist was all smiles as I met her that morning of the 13th March 2006. She confirmed I was all clear, and would need six-monthly check-ups for the first two years and thereafter yearly check –ups. My first check up was scheduled for 16th October and I would need a blood test a month before that where TSH and thyroglobulin levels would be checked again. As long as the TSH was kept suppressed with the correct amount of Thyroxine and the thyroglobulin level under 2, the cancer would hopefully not return. After a clean scan, if the thyroglobulin level started to rise, it would be assumed that more thyroid cancer cells were growing. I said I was feeling fine on 150mcg of Thyroxine without too many side-effects. I only occasionally felt hot, and could hear my heart pounding in my ears only if I bent forward. She decided to keep me on 150mcg for the time being. I could also now go ahead with the jaw operation, and decided to ask the Oral Surgeon if that could be booked in for July 2006. Hopefully after this I would need no more operations.

I toyed with the idea of finally telling my mother that I had had thyroid cancer but was now all clear, but I decided to go along with the 'ignorance is bliss' theory. That would have worked but after having submitted my story to a press agency, there was a chance it could be published (it wasn't). I had to tell her before the nation read about it. She took it better than I'd expected actually. Because she'd had cancer herself and survived, she understood you don't automatically die just because you've been diagnosed with the disease. She had wondered if it was cancer, but hadn't liked to ask.

Also, after the usual long wait on the NHS, the Speech Therapist contacted me in March to ask if I still needed an appointment. As my voice had improved dramatically, I did not think an appointment was necessary, so she said she would send me information in the post of how to look after my voice. I still had the option of surgery in the future, but did not think any speech therapy would make a huge difference.

71

CHAPTER SEVENTEEN – EMPTY NEST

I had decided that having cancer was not altogether a negative experience. It had improved my career prospects for a start. It had also made me re-define my priorities in life. I now did not worry about much at all – things in the past that would have caused me sleepless nights now did not bother me. As long as you have your health and a loving family, nothing else matters. I also counted each new day as a bonus because had the 'multinodular goitre' been left untreated, I would most probably not have survived much past my 50th birthday.

Also I realised that Doctors are not infallible and can sometimes make misdiagnoses. The Radiologist who had given me the ultrasound scan a year before and had diagnosed the 'multinodular goitre' was quite a respected Consultant in the hospital where I work, and also one of its Directors. His scan report had been sent to the Endocrinologist who had probably based his findings on it, and consequently no alarm bells had rung straight away. It was a good thing I had decided myself to have the lump surgically removed, as four years down the line I am still here, but who is to say I would have been if the lump had been left alone?

The only cloud on my now bright horizon was that Matthew announced he would be leaving home to share a rented house with Anna and some of Anna's friends who were all studying music at Homerton College, Cambridge. He would start looking for work local to the college. They were going to view a 5-bedroomed house in Cherry Hinton Road on Saturday March 11th 2006. The last bird was fleeing the nest and I knew I would definitely have the 'Empty Nest Syndrome'. Although Matt was more often out than at home, I always knew he would be returning at some point for his dinner and a chat and I would have to get used to not seeing him so often. His brother had moved out three years previously and I had slowly got used to his absence, but it would be much different with no boys in the house at all. I had nightmare visions of wandering the house looking for my elusive children.

Matt phoned home very excited later on that day. They had decided to take the tenancy of the house, and could move in any time from July 1st onwards. My nightmare would soon be a reality. It's only now when faced with an empty nest that I realise what my own mother, a widow at the time, must have gone through when her only child, me, decided to leave home. My father had died the year previously in 1977, and I had jumped ship aged 20 as soon as I could find somebody to share a flat with. In the long run it helped her though, as she learned to drive, bought a car, took herself dancing and found new friends and even a boyfriend for a while. Perhaps with all this new-found freedom, I would be able to learn to ski, salsa, abseil or whatever - the world was mine for the taking! It made no difference at first – I pined and pined for my little boy. I gradually came to realise (as does every mother) that I was pining for his lost childhood and because I was not needed any more now that my little boy was a fully grown man. Of course I knew Matt was entitled to a life of his own, but it's not something that a mother can get used to straight away. It took a year or so for me to become used to his absence, and I'm sure Matthew and Anna are very happy that I did. Our children are only loaned to us for a short time, and we must let them go when they are ready.

CHAPTER EIGHTEEN - SECONDARIES

Fast forward a few months. Matt had settled with Anna in the house in Cherry Hinton Road, Cambridge, and would be joined by the other four students towards the end of September. He had found engineering work in nearby Sawston, and was enjoying the challenge of being given a new type of CNC lathe to work on. There would be promotion for him and a pay rise in 2007 when he had mastered it and its programming complexities. Phil and I (well, Phil was anyway) were slowly getting used to just the two of us in the house, but were still following the band around to gigs. Matt had joined a new band when he left for Cambridge. This band were more focused, more musically competent, and certainly looked as if they might be going places. Lee and Sarah were happy and little Sophie was beginning to crawl about. I had had an arthroscopy of my left jaw joint done in late July under a general anaesthetic at the Nuffield hospital at Ipswich, but unfortunately I knew the operation had not been a success. In fact the joint was worse than ever, locking during the day, locking whilst eating, locking all night, and making a horrible clicking noise every time I opened my mouth. To top it all, after the arthroscopy I was only allowed to eat pureed food for six weeks to give the joint a chance to heal. The kitchen staff in the hospital at work were very kind and made me a pureed lunch every day, but I couldn't understand why I was feeling queasy every day about two hours after eating it. On further discussion with the kitchen staff, I found out they were putting fortified milk powder in the soup (I have a really bad milk intolerance) and I was having to pull over to the side of the road on the way home every day because I felt so sick!

The Oral Surgeon said more invasive surgery was needed that would correct the problem. I needed a meniscectomy – removal of the meniscus disc in the joint. He hadn't wanted to do that first off as he had hoped the keyhole arthroscopy to remove debris and scar tissue would have sufficed. I did not fancy any more anaesthetics and surgery at that time, so decided to put it off until the new year. A week or so before the arthroscopy I had also had a temporary crown put on the troublesome back tooth that was cracked. It was September before the actual crown could be put on, as the arthroscopy had caused me to be unable to open my mouth properly for six weeks, so the Dentist could not have fitted the permanent crown properly before then. This delay caused an infection in the temporary crown that would not go away.

Also in September it was time for me to get a blood test done, so the results would be ready for my six-month check-up with the Oncologist at The Nuffield hospital, Cambridge. I thought I may as well get the blood test done whilst at work, so quickly popped down to Pathology early on 4th September 2006. I knew the thyroglobulin test would take some time to come back, so decided to put the result to the back of my mind for a month or so. I was all-clear anyway, so I assumed the result would be 2 or lower. I actually forgot about checking the result until the day before Phil and I were to leave for a week's holiday at the usual Isle of Wight bungalow at the end of September. No Doctor had been in touch with the result. I actually asked a colleague at work to look up the result. It came back 10.2.

The holiday was spoilt for me, as I knew the cancer had come back. The result should have been 2 or under, and here it was staring me in the face at 10.2. (when the thyroid cancer was first diagnosed, the thyroglobulin had been 78 which had dropped to 4.9 after the first RAI dose). The night before we went away, I hurriedly emailed my Oncologist (who had not received a copy of the result so was uninformed) to let her know the outcome. Back came the reply almost at once to bring forward my appointment to see her as soon as we were back from the Isle of Wight.

I spent the whole week's holiday worried sick but trying not to show it so as not to worry Phil. I expect he was just as worried but did not want to alarm me, so we dutifully did not talk about it much and carried on as though everything was all right. At my appointment at the Cambridge Nuffield on October 2nd, the Oncologist ordered another blood test and a CT scan of the neck and chest to check for secondaries. The blood test at the Nuffield would be sent to Cardiff to be assessed, which was a different destination to where the blood test at the Pathology laboratory at work had been sent to. I was scanned, had blood taken, and went home to worry.

Having heard nothing after a couple of weeks, I emailed the Oncologist to ask if any secondaries had been found on the CT scan. Almost immediately she phoned me to say that she and the Radiologist had been poring over my scans all afternoon, and unfortunately they could see small secondary spots on the lungs. Yes it was 'disappointing' that this had happened, and I would need another dose of Radioactive Iodine to hopefully put it right. This time I would have to come off my Thyroxine tablets beforehand to ensure the treatment would be effective. This put the idea in my mind that perhaps the second treatment with the Thyrogen had not been as effective as becoming hypo, and had caused the cancer to spread. She told me that many patients with secondary thyroid cancer were still alive 30+ years later, as being slightly over-medicated on Thyroxine suppressed the thyroid stimulating hormone and stopped the lung secondaries from growing. She would book me into the RadioIodine Suite at Addenbrooke's for another ablative dose in the near future. She also mentioned the latest thyroglobulin result was 0.5. I could not understand the discrepancy, and made a mental note to ask her why on my next appointment on December 4th. I put the phone down and broke the news to Phil, and we both sat looking at each other with tears in our eyes. We knew it was serious this time – the cancer had spread to the lungs. I told him if and when I was terminal and my body could not take any more, that I wanted to go to the Dignitas clinic in Switzerland where they practiced euthanasia as I did not want to suffer. He looked as devastated as I felt.

Meanwhile I had to go back to work and tell everybody that I now had secondaries and would need a month off work for more treatment. I would need to switch back to T3's for a month, and then stop taking any Thyroxine tablets at all for two weeks prior to the start of my treatment on December 11th. I would become 'hypo' again. I remembered the aching legs, the puffy face and tired eyes and felt very depressed for the first time in a long time. Everyone at work was very kind, but I hated being different. I wanted to be normal and to do what everybody else did; to get up, go to work, come home and cook dinner etc. – not the constant round of hospital visits and Doctors' surgeries. News quickly spread around the workplace (a hospital grapevine is very efficient) and I was suddenly the talk of the office. I told my Manager that my last day at work would be Friday 24th of November, because on the following Monday I would be taking no Thyroxine tablets and would feel too tired to work. I would not be back at work until Tuesday January 2nd 2007.

I also decided to ask the original Endocrinologist who saw me in December 2004 for my notes and ultrasound scan reports. I wanted them to refer to as I was in the process of writing this book. I rang him at home after a few emails had produced nothing. He was worried there was going to be a complaint, but could hardly refuse me the notes as they were mine anyway. Eventually a couple of weeks later the notes arrived but not the ultrasound reports, as he informed me that the Radiologist would have to give his permission for me to have them. After consulting with colleagues and confirming that I was entitled to have them, they were eventually faxed to me from the Bury Nuffield after some interjection by a senior work colleague.

October 2006 saw me moping around the house and trying to be cheerful at work, but feeling desperately sad. I felt my life was to be cut short and I was not ready to die. I wanted to see my granddaughter grow up, to see how the boys' jobs progressed, and I wanted to see how Matt's band fared. They had already won a band competition locally after only two months of playing together, and they showed so much promise. I realised I had inherited the cancer gene from one or both parents, and wondered if I was going to die at the same early age as my father. By the time he was my age, he only had a few months left of life.

One morning at work I was pushing my trolley of medical notes down to Medical Records. My chin was down and I felt that trying to carry on a normal life was meaningless when I was going to die anyway. What was the point? I had been to the medical library and looked up secondary thyroid cancer. Survival rates were as low as 50%. With cumulative doses of Radioactive Iodine, there was a chance of getting leukaemia as well if you had had more than 18,500 bequerels (I had had about 9000 so far). But as I pushed the trolley down the corridor, I was suddenly overcome with a strange feeling that somehow everything was going to be ok. I suddenly felt lighter in mood and did not know why. It was only sometime later that I realised the feeling I experienced was when I was walking past the chapel. I am not in any way religious and cannot give any explanation for it, but in the depths of my misery I wondered if by a miracle I was going to survive. Back at home I called out for some sort of sign that I would be ok (I do believe in the spirit world and have received messages from many Mediums proving there is a spirit world). My call was answered within a very short time by a lightbulb popping out of its socket in the electric fire, which it had never done before. The bulb was still working when Phil put it back in. When lying awake in bed one night, I opened my eyes to put the light on to get a drink, and there was somebody sitting on the edge of my bed smiling. She had a white coat on and she looked like my Oncologist. She stayed there for a couple of seconds before disappearing.

I clutched at straws. These were signs. I was going to be ok. I decided to book my menisectomy operation for the period prior to coming off the Thyroxine tablets so that I would only need to take one lot of sick leave and hopefully all my problems would be sorted at the same time. I was suddenly infused with hope. I explained all to the Oral Surgeon who could see I was still fit and said it would not be a problem to do the operation (the Oncologist had also said it would be ok). He would book me in for Thursday 23rd November 2006 at the Nuffield hospital at Ipswich. I asked him to take the troublesome crowned tooth out as well, which had become a huge abscess. Bacteria had got in whilst the temporary crown was on, and no antibiotic would touch it. He agreed, and I said a temporary goodbye to my work colleagues on Wednesday 22nd November. I hoped I felt recovered enough from the menisectomy before I stopped the Thyroxine T3 tablets on Monday November 27th.

CHAPTER NINETEEN – MENISCECTOMY OF LEFT JAW

Thursday November 23rd saw Phil and I waiting in room 6 at the Ipswich Nuffield for my operation. Unfortunately I was last on the list (as usual) because I was the 'tricky' one. When the Nurse had come in to take my temperature, she informed me it was high. I tried to tell her it was sometimes on the high side due to being over-medicated on Thyroxine, but I was sure she thought I had an infection. The Anaesthetist had been to see me and had been informed of my locking jaw, secondary lung cancer, and the tendency for my heart rate and blood pressure to rise considerably after procedures involving a general anaesthetic. I imagined him throwing up his hands in horror and running away. He looked at my previous anaesthetic chart from July, but could see no real problems as the blood pressure and heart rate always settle down once I am asleep. He seemed very calm and confident and his attitude helped me to remain relatively calm. Perhaps I was not too much of a freak after all. Matt telephoned during the morning, but I could not tell him much as I was still waiting.

Finally at noon I was informed Theatre was ready for me. I dutifully got into bed in my gown and anti-DVT stockings, and hoped for the best. In the anaesthetic room a cannula was put in my hand and a sedative injected into it. A blanket came down over my brain and I remember no more until waking up in Recovery about an hour and a half later. I could hear somebody saying that I was 'tachycardic' but I remember thinking that I usually am after operations anyway. There was a swab in my mouth catching any remaining blood from the tooth extraction (thank goodness I had finally seen the last of lower right seven) and what felt like a very tight turban on my head with something hanging off of it. I asked for a drink but was refused as it was too soon. I was told that now I was awake I could be taken back to my room.

Dear Phil was waiting yet again for me to come back. I wanted to feel what was hanging off the turban, but he put my hand down and said it was just a drain held in place by bandages (so that was what the turban was). It hurt to try and open my mouth, so I thought it best not to try. The Nurse asked if I was in any pain, but thinking about it, it only hurt when I opened my mouth, so I said I didn't need any painkillers as the pain was not constant. Everybody seemed amazed. I was hoping I did not become nauseous, as it would be excruciatingly painful to be sick. I had remembered to ask the Anaesthetist for a good anti-sickness injection and it seemed to have done the trick.

Phil gave me sips of water. I slowly came round and was thankful it was all over. Phil helped me to the toilet (what more could you want from a husband!) and I slowly started moving about. Now I just needed to recover enough before the RadioIodine treatment in a couple of weeks' time.

I was discharged the next day after the Nurse had taken the drain and cannula out, and had taken the turban off (what a relief to be free from that). There was a long scar going from just in front of my ear and up into my hairline. My hair had been shaved above my ear, and that was the worst bit as far as I was concerned! I had lots of stitches that would need taking out on Tuesday December 5th (my next appointment with the Oral Surgeon). I had a red rash on my face and chest that appeared in the car going home, but I knew that was the effect of the anaesthetic so did not worry about that too much. After my thyroidectomy, my face had changed to a brown colour and little rashes had appeared and disappeared, so I knew it was my body objecting to the anaesthetic in the only way it knew how. I did not know if the operation had been a success as it would probably be a week or so before I could open my mouth (if the last jaw operation was anything to go by), but I had a feeling this time the operation would work. Before I left the hospital the Surgeon informed me he had never seen a disc so shredded. I had excelled myself in the realms of meniscus maceration.

Matt turned 21 during my recovery period. There was a party arranged at Cambridge on Saturday 25th November, but I did not feel well enough to go. Phil attended and said it all went off very well. I would have to wait for Anna's parents' New Year's Eve party instead. It looked to be a good night. I would be in charge of the music, and there would be fireworks at midnight in the garden. Evening dress was essential. I couldn't wait. It would be a chance to wear the expensive evening dress I had bought for the Caribbean cruise the year before. I would have to get my hairdresser to try and cut my hair so the two sides above my ears looked equal. At the moment it was rather lopsided; I was bald on one side and normal on the other.

After a week of recovery, I knew the operation had worked. There was no loud clicking when I opened my mouth, and my jaw had stopped locking. It had all been worth it. Awesome. I didn't even mind another six weeks of pureed food again, because this time I could see an end to it all. The kitchen staff went out of their way this time not to give me anything with milk powder in it, and I was fine.

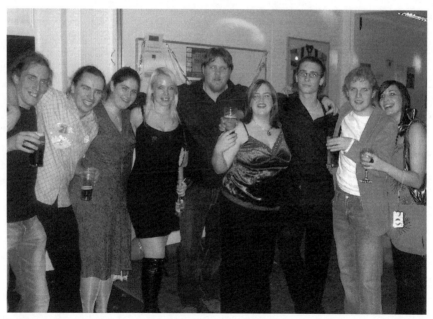

Matt's 21st birthday party (Matt 2nd from left with band members & girlfriends)

CHAPTER TWENTY – THIRD RADIOACTIVE IODINE TREATMENT

I had an appointment with the Oncologist on Monday 4th December. By then I had been hypo for a week and was feeling cold (very unusual for me!) tired, and achey. I had also picked up what I thought was a slight chest infection from somewhere. The Oncologist really couldn't tell me the outcome of the RAI treatment – whether it would kill the secondaries or not. I suppose she didn't know herself. All she could tell me was that she knew some patients where it had worked (she presumably knew of patients where it had not worked, but was not saying). Apparently the secondaries did not usually grow if they were suppressed with enough Thyroxine. She had checked with eminent London Oncologists as to my treatment, and had been reassured that everything was being done that could be done. Apparently I was making thyroglobulin antibodies which complicated matters somewhat (about 20% of thyroid cancer patients do this). My personal marker which would show either the cure or advancement of my cancer was to be the amount of thyroglobulin antibodies in my blood, and not the amount of thyroglobulin. The thyroglobulin result of 10.2 had been sent from the processing laboratories at Birmingham, and usually my Oncologist would have sent it off to the laboratories at Cardiff. She said different laboratories either overestimated or underestimated the result. She said a result from Cardiff would have been lower. I would be having another blood test the following week in the RAI room before the start of the treatment, and presumably another one at a later date, and a scan at the end of the week as usual when the radiation levels in my body were at a safe dose. Hopefully the spots on my lungs would show up on the scanner, which meant they had taken up the RAI. We made another appointment for me to come back on 15th January 2007 for the results of the scan and blood tests. I decided I wasn't going to worry about it all over Christmas – what will be will be. What I was looking forward to was the next day (Tuesday 5th December) when the stitches in my jaw were due to come out. I had an appointment with the Oral Surgeon at 2.25pm.

After my stitches had come out on the Tuesday, I started feeling quite ill with what I thought was a chest infection. Because I was hypothyroid, the phlegm was so thick and slow moving, that on a couple of occasions it had lodged in my windpipe preventing me from breathing in properly. I had had to try and take a big breath in and cough it up. It was very scary, and I didn't think I would be well enough to have the RadioIodine dose. I phoned the Oncologist on the Friday and she suggested I come into Addenbrooke's and have some tests to check for infection. My heart sank. Surely I hadn't taken all this time off work and got this far to be told it wasn't going to happen?

Phil and I arrived at the RadioIodine Suite on the Friday evening 8th December. The Oncologist had arranged a chest x-ray and blood tests for me, and the Nurses put me on antibiotics and a nebuliser at regular intervals. She also had the ENT Surgeon who I had seen regarding my voice to look down my throat and see if all was well. He couldn't see anything too untoward, just lots of secretions going down the back of the nose. The blood results came back that it wasn't a chest infection and that I would be well enough to undergo the treatment. Just being hypo had slowed down the phlegm production (as indeed it slows everything else down as well), but it was making me feel quite unwell in the process. I stayed in for five nights eventually, and had my treatment on the Monday morning. During the Monday night I felt quite sick and panicked that I might vomit and injure my jaw. I quickly popped an anti-sickness pill and thankfully the feeling wore off. I wondered how much more my body could cope with. It really was turning out to be a massive endurance exercise. Also my eyes were not focusing due to being hypo – as if I needed any more things wrong with me.

By the Wednesday the Radioactive Iodine levels were low enough for me to go home. I hobbled out of Ward A5 and wondered how I was going to stay awake long enough to get to the car. I'd had no proper sleep since arriving at Addenbrooke's due to the phlegm problem, and also due to the bed being very uncomfortable. During the ride home I drifted in and out of sleep and worried about having to lie flat for the scan on the Friday, as it would be quite uncomfortable with the amount of phlegm at the back of my throat. The Physicist had mentioned my worries to the scan Technicians, and they apparently would do their best to accommodate me. They could do the scan in sections so that I could be propped up. As it turned out, they did not even ask me if I wanted propping up; they just left me to get on with it and use mind over matter. It was a most uncomfortable 15 – 20 minutes.

My legs did not recover as quickly after re-starting the Thyroxine as they had the first time. It took a good week for the achy calves to go, and for me to be able to stay awake for any length of time. I was determined to enjoy Christmas and not worry about if the treatment had worked or not. I hoped that after all I had suffered it would work, but secretly had doubts.

CHAPTER TWENTY-ONE – AFTERMATH OF TREATMENT

Christmas Eve saw Phil, Mum, and I at Anna's parents' house for a get-together. The Thyroxine levels were slowly coming up again and I was feeling a little better. The phlegm problem was still there, but at least it wasn't catching in my windpipe any more. Christmas Day lunch was in the Spread Eagle in Bury St Edmunds with Matt, Anna and Mum. Lee, Sarah and Sophie came to see us in the afternoon to exchange presents. There was some good news – I was going to be a grandmother again. Baby number 2 was due 27th August 2007! Lee also joined us for lunch on 28th December at The Rushbrooke Arms in Sicklesmere when Mary, Dave, and Jenny came for a visit.

It was a great New Year's Eve party at Anna's parents' house. I danced until midnight and then felt really tired and wanted to go home. We had some gatecrashers who came in the front door, did a conga around the room, and then disappeared out the back door into the garden never to be seen again. Goodness knows where they went.

I was on tenterhooks when my appointment with the Oncologist came around on January 15th. I told Phil I wanted to go on my own. I didn't want to put him through any more upset in case it was bad news.

No uptake was shown on the Gamma scan. The Oncologist explained that it probably meant that the spots were too small to show up. I secretly thought it probably meant that the treatment hadn't worked, but decided to go along with her explanation as it offered more hope. She said she was going to give the radioactive Iodine a few months to work, then I would need another blood test in May to check thyroglobulin antibody levels, and then another CT scan in early June to see if the spots were still there. Another appointment was made with her for July 2nd to obtain the results. It would mean another six months of waiting, but there was no other way round it. I came away disappointed and frustrated at the long wait to find out if I was going to be cured or not.

The phlegm problem persisted and would not go away (I had been told that there had been uptake of radiation in the back of my nose – hence the cause of the problem). My salivary glands became sore and painful during March and both problems carried on through spring and summer. The ENT Surgeon prescribed a nasal spray and some pills to thin out the phlegm. It worked slightly and the phlegm became a little thinner, but unfortunately did not dry up completely. My mouth and throat were constantly dry due to the salivary glands not working properly, and I had to sip water all day, which eased the problem. I carried on at work but became tired of being asked the eternal question 'When will you be getting your results'? People were either trying to be kind and caring, or were just nosey – I couldn't decide which.

CHAPTER TWENTY-TWO – RESULT OF CT SCAN

It was a wonder the whole of the Nuffield Hospital couldn't hear my heart beating as I sat in the Oncologist's office in July to hear my results. She said she could not see any lung secondaries on the scan, but sometimes it was difficult to see them if they were very small, and there were two small nodules in the lungs that hadn't changed from the previous scan. She also said that the scan showed two enlarged lymph nodes in my neck, which had got bigger since the first CT scan. She had not mentioned them the previous time, as she wanted to wait to see if the lung secondaries had enlarged. If they had not, then it would be worth giving me an operation (a left-sided neck dissection) to remove the lymph nodes. If the lung secondaries had become larger, then it would not have been worth putting me through the operation as I would have been terminal. So, at least I knew I was not terminal, but I would rather have been kept informed of my condition. She told me the ENT Surgeon who I had been seeing for my lack of voice and for the phlegm problem would do the neck dissection. I would receive an appointment to see him in the post. Swings and roundabouts – life gives with one hand and takes away with the other. I felt pleased that the lung spots had not enlarged, but disappointed that I would have to have yet another operation. I thought hard and decided it would be a good idea to have the operation at the end of August. Then I would be recovered before Phil and I had our joint 50th birthday celebration party on October 13th, and then also I would be able to enjoy our holiday to St Lucia in November. There were also some music festivals mid –August which Matt's band were due to play in, and we had already booked tickets for these. Matt had also secured a better job with Marshall Aerospace in Cambridge which paid him another £9,000 per year. I was also due to become a Granny again as Sarah's caesarean was due on 14th August. They had chosen the name Caitlin Marie for the new baby. I told the ENT surgeon that I would be ready for the operation on August 30th. By then there would be nothing left to look forward to except a Rush concert on October 6th. I sat in the car with Phil afterwards and cried.

The days passed slowly. Baby Caitlin being born helped to divert my thoughts for a while. The operation seemed to be on my mind the whole time. I wondered how the phlegm problem would affect me during the op; whether it would catch in my windpipe when I was unconscious. I resolved to mention the problem to the Anaesthetist on the day. Food also seemed to get stuck sometimes, but a way round this problem I found was to eat slower and have smaller mouthfuls.

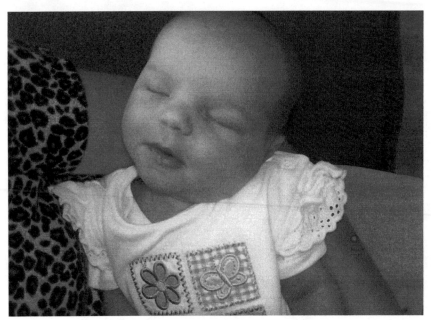

Baby Caitlin Marie born 14/8/07

CHAPTER TWENTY-THREE – NECK DISSECTION

Thursday 30th August came around far too quickly. Phil drove me to the Cambridge Nuffield, and we arrived about 12.30. The staff seemed very kind and helpful. I was given the usual gown and TED stockings to put on, and was told my operation would be at about 3pm. I was visited by the Anaesthetist and I told him of the phlegm problem. He didn't seem to think this mattered and said he would 'look after me'. The Surgeon came to see me beforehand too to take my consent and list all the things that could go wrong (pain, bleeding, infection, numbness, frozen shoulder, abnormal tongue movement, and difficulty in swallowing), and I mentioned the phlegm problem again. I had also visited the Thyroid Cancer Support group online and had been reading the latest messages. One person who had had a neck dissection also had my voice box problem. When she vomited after the operation, the aspirant went down the windpipe and she had spent three days coughing it up. I had not vomited since before the original thyroidectomy, so had no idea if this would happen to me. The Surgeon reassured me and said this was unlikely. If my throat had been open that much, then food and drink would go down the windpipe as well. I thought about it and was slightly reassured. There were also the usual visits from the Doctor to put the cannula in, and one of the nursing staff to admit me and go through my medications.

Finally it was time to go. I actually walked with a Nurse and Phil to the Theatre at 3pm. There I was met by the Anaesthetist. I laid down on the trolley and said goodbye to Phil. I felt the anaesthetic go into the cannula and up my arm, then do not remember any more until waking up rather groggy in Recovery. I remember feeling extremely hot, and heard the Nurse saying that I was tachycardic. It's the usual problem I get after operations – the heart rate and blood pressure go up for a couple of days. I was also aware that my heels hurt very much from laying flat for a length of time on the operating table.

As soon as I was awake, I was taken back to my room. Phil had been rather worried as I had been gone for about six hours. The Surgeon came in to say that he had taken all the lymphatic tissue out on the left hand side of the neck (the right side at that time had been unaffected), and that after he had finished he could not see anything sinister left on that side in the neck. He said there had been a number of enlarged lymph glands, and also a very enlarged one down in the old thyroid bed which were now all gone. He said I might need some more Radioactive Iodine to kill any stray cells, and also the right side of the neck may or may not need attention in the future. I asked why the radiation the previous December had not killed all these glands, and the Surgeon said that was because they were too big (the radiation works better on small pieces of tissue). I had two drains in, and would not be allowed home until these had been taken out. There was a big waterproof dressing covering the front of my neck and up to my left ear. I felt surprised to be still alive and that no phlegm had gone down the windpipe.

Over the next couple of days I tried to get out of bed. At first poor old Phil had to bring the bedpans in again, as they had inserted another cannula in Theatre for fluids and I was weeing for England again. Once again he did not shirk his duties, and hurried back and forth emptying them. On the second day I managed to get out of bed and use the commode which was an improvement on the bedpans. My back hurt, and on looking, Phil could see there was a graze which had not been there before the operation. Very mysterious! The Nurse dressed it and reported it to Matron.

I was glad that I still had my coughing mechanism, which had been lacking after the thyroidectomy. The phlegm after that operation was much worse than this one, as I had not been able to cough it up. I had a couple of nebulisers as suggested by the Nurse, but this time it did not seem too bad. The only thing I noticed on the second day was a tingling in my hands and face and tongue. I wondered if my parathyroid glands had been affected, but the Doctor said wait and see if things settled down first. On the third day the tingling went, so that was a relief. The reversing agent that I had been given in Theatre to wake me up stayed in my system for quite a few days after. Every time

I nodded off to sleep, then my brain woke me up straight away, as had happened with the thyroidectomy. It was awful.

On the Saturday one of the drains was taken out and the remaining one the day after. I was allowed to go home on the Sunday to recover. The Nurse changed the dressing before I left, and said not to be too shocked at all the staples in my neck when I saw them. When Phil put a clean dressing on at home, he also told me not to look at the wound until all the staples were out. I decided to hold him to this, and therefore had no idea how it looked, but it must have looked bad.

Secretly I did look though, when Phil had gone back to work the next week and I was left at home to recover. I pulled the dressing back and yes it did look hideous, but I thought at the time how neat all the staples looked, stretching in a long line from my ear down to the middle of my neck. This Surgeon knew his business, I thought. I was rather glad all the skin was numb surrounding the scar, because then it wouldn't hurt too much when the staples were all taken out on the following Thursday. I seemed to be in continual pain in an area just below the scar on my chest. My neck and shoulder were stiff and sore and the skin was numb to the touch; indeed I couldn't move my head to the left at all. My left shoulder felt as though the Surgeon had cut a big gouge along the top of it and then left it open and raw. When Phil took me to the GP surgery to have the staples removed, the Nurse noticed the scar looked a bit red and called the Doctor to have a look at it. The Doctor agreed and put me on an antibiotic just to make sure it did not become too infected.

The pain was still there (although a little less) when I went to see the Surgeon three weeks later for my check-up. He said there was nothing to worry about – I was bound to be in pain and it, plus the numbness, would go in time. He stressed I had to move my neck as much as I could otherwise it could become permanently stiff. He said results of the biopsy showed that 25 lymph glands had been removed and the majority of them had been cancerous, but at the end of the operation he had not seen any sinister-looking lymph nodes left. I would need another CT scan in three months' time to check there were not any enlarged glands left, and lifelong follow-up scans thereafter. He did not think the Radioactive Iodine worked on me particularly well, so it would have to be surgery in the future for any suspicious lumps that arose. He thought I would have a normal lifespan, but this type of cancer, although slow-growing, could come back at any time and therefore I might need more surgery. He checked my voice box with the camera just to make sure that my right vocal cord was still working: it was!

CHAPTER TWENTY-FOUR – I MADE IT TO 50 AGAINST ALL ODDS!

Altogether I was off work for five weeks. It was a bigger operation than the original thyroidectomy, so took a little longer to recover from. The Surgeon did say that it would take about six to nine months for the numbness to go, so I returned to work still feeling numb and a bit sore. I still had to cope with the phlegm problem as well, but it was not as bad as it had been earlier in the year. Also my eyes had been affected by the previous year's radiation and were watery and often infected. I had to carry Fucithalmic eye ointment around all the time.

Fortunately I was still able to enjoy the joint 50th birthday party that I had organised for Phil and myself on October 13th, one week after my return to work. I had a lovely time and danced for most of the night. I had made it to 50. I was very happy being surrounded with family and friends, and it made a lovely change from hospitals and Doctors. My cousin Phillip had even come over from Saudi Arabia for the occasion, and made us a huge cake, which could have fed the entire village. The week after that was another party to celebrate Anna's 21st birthday. This time Phil had to dress in his dinner suit, and I had had to scour the shops to find a 20's flapper dress, as the party had a 20's theme. Again I danced most of the night. I was partying for England even though I still couldn't move my neck very well. A couple of weeks after this Phil and I flew to St. Lucia for a well earned holiday. We stayed at the Sandals resort in Halcyon Bay in Castries. The sun shone, we lazed on the beach, and my scar healed slowly. It was bliss.

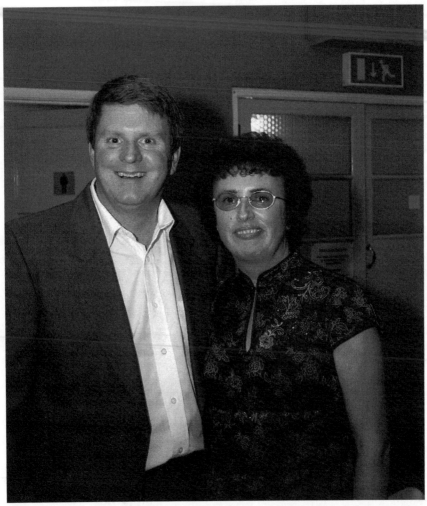

Phil and I at our joint 50th birthday party – October 2007. I searched through my wardrobe to try and find a high-collared top to cover the scar up on the night.

Back at home in December it was time for the three month scan. The skin surrounding the scar was still numb. The CT scan itself was not too bad – the only part I didn't like was when the dye was injected. It made me feel very hot, but did not last for too long. Also part of the process of scanning the neck and chest involved holding my breath which wasn't too pleasant either, but I could cope with that.

Two weeks after the scan on December 17th I faced the ENT surgeon who had performed the neck dissection. My heart was racing in dread of the possible results. He was smiling so it couldn't be too bad. There were a couple of tiny nodes which he was going to keep an eye on, but all in all it wasn't too bad. The nodules in the lungs still hadn't changed, and he wasn't sure whether there was an enlarged lymph gland near my left ear, or whether it was muscle tissue. As far as I could tell, it was a case of looking at the next CT scan results in a year's time to see if anything changed and if so, where they went from there, and to take another blood sample to see if the thyroglobulin antibodies had reduced any. At least I didn't need any more operations in the near future, and I still wasn't terminal. Oh well, at least I could enjoy Christmas!

This year we were all invited for Christmas dinner at Anna's parents' house in Ipswich. We provided the turkey and it was lovely sitting round a big table on Christmas Day with Matt, Anna, and all her family. They even invited my mother to share in the celebrations. Boxing Day saw everyone at our house for a get-together, and then it was back to Anna's parents on New Year's Eve for a party to see in 2008. Perhaps it would be next year when I would be finally rid of this dreadful disease.

CHAPTER TWENTY-FIVE - 2008

2008 started off with a visit in early January to London Theatreland to see Phantom of the Opera. I loved it so much that I vowed to go again before too long.

I also decided to make an appointment at the Eye Clinic at the hospital where I worked to find out why my eyes were always watery and why they often became infected. I was told I had blepharitis, an inflammation of the eyelids, and this was probably not caused by the radioactive Iodine as I had first thought. I was told to wash the eyes thoroughly with hot water every morning and evening, which would help to clear any dirt and debris, the likely causes of this irritating condition. Strangely enough this did seem to help a little bit, but did not take away the problem altogether.

January 2008 was also the time when I decided to enrich my mind and began to learn Pitman 2000 shorthand. Eight months later I still had not progressed very far, but it did stretch my middle-aged mind trying to remember all the little lines, dots, and squiggles. I also signed on at work for an NVQ Level 3 in Business Admin. It was all free and so why not?

On February 18th it was time for another check-up with the ENT surgeon who had performed my neck dissection. I still had no feeling on the left side of my neck, and if I faced frontwards and moved my head over to the right, it felt very peculiar indeed. Still, the scar had healed well, and he couldn't detect any new lumps or bumps in my neck, which was all to the good. I still had phlegm problems at the back of my throat, and sometimes food became stuck if I did not eat carefully, but on the whole things were improving. He said the blood test performed in December did show a slight reduction in thyroglobulin, but it was not really worth me having further blood tests as the antibodies I made rendered tests mostly non-viable. They would concentrate mainly on the results of CT scans to plan further treatment. It seemed that radioactive Iodine was not very successful either, so as far as I could see only surgery would be available to me as a treatment should the cancer progress. Another check-up was due three months hence, and another scan was due in December. I felt well enough, was enjoying work, and also was relieved no further surgery was needed at that time. Phil and I had a nice week off work in March and visited Old Trafford football ground for a tour (part of Phil's Christmas present from me), and had a boat ride up the Thames from Greenwich culminating in a ride on the London Eye.

I had decided just before Christmas it was time for me to again try to stop the Norethisterone tablets that regulated my periods and had thankfully eradicated my PMT problems for the past 12 years. I was 50 now and surely I must be pre-menopausal? All my old schoolfriends were going through the menopause, as I had found out when we attended their 50th birthday dinners in April and May. A few months off the tablets to get the Norethisterone out of my system and then a blood test would show whether I should consider HRT or not. I didn't feel menopausal though, and by February it was clear that coming off the tablets was giving me some 'interesting' side effects (but we won't go there). It was no good though – the terrible PMT symptoms had returned by May, and I couldn't wait to have the blood test done and start taking the tablets again. The blood test showed normal levels. I was not menopausal, so before you could say 'hot flushes' I was back on the Norethisterone tablets. The GP assured me that I would know when I was menopausal as Norethisterone is progesterone only, so the tablets would not stop the dreaded hot flushes when they occurred, only oestrogen would do that. It was a terrible mistake coming off the Norethisterone, as my body seemed to produce too much oestrogen and I did not seem to have the progesterone to counterbalance it. I must be the only middle aged woman in the world who is actually looking forward to the menopause. I try and get by without taking tablets if at all possible, but Norethisterone and Thyroxine are the two I cannot do without!

The blood test had also shown that my eosinophil count was raised. I quickly contacted my Oncologist, who assured me that as I suffered from hayfever and it was the hayfever season, this was the reason that the eosinophil count had risen to 1.7. She asked me to have another blood test in August after the hayfever season had finished, to see if it had decreased any. I was reassured by this, as I had read on the internet that it could be a sign of leukaemia. Perhaps I read too much.

May 2008 was also the time that Matt and Anna found a place of their own. They moved into rented accommodation in Cherry Hinton, and seemed extremely happy together. They had tired of sharing a house with five other students. Two of the students had very strange habits, would not talk to the others, and would share a bath at 2am. These two eventually married, but not before Matt and Anna had moved out. With a place of their own, Anna could at last have the parlourgrand piano that had belonged to her grandfather taken out of storage and deposited in their front room. Matt had one of the bedrooms as his music room, with all his amps and guitars set up to his liking. He was as happy as a pig wallowing in the brown stuff.

Another successful check up with the ENT Surgeon occurred in May. There was nothing much to report. No lumps could be felt in my neck. He said the Oncologist wanted to see me in August for a check-up, and then it would be back to him again in November for another check up.

I also visited a world-famous Healer at his home near Bury St Edmunds in May for the first of three healing sessions. He placed his hands on my neck for about 20 minutes to the accompaniment of soothing music. I had read that it had been scientifically proven that the force of his healing hands could change cancer cells in test tubes, and he had cured many people with cancer, including his own wife. If it worked I was all for it. I was doing all I could to help myself.

We were getting out and about with a couple of friends from work to see various bands. Matt's band were winding down after a very successful 2007, where they had played at a couple of big festivals. Two band members were leaving to go to University, and one band member left because he was fed up with it all. Phil and I bought tickets for the

Isle of Wight Festival which was due to be held in June, and asked the lovely Betty if we could rent her bungalow again so that we didn't have to suffer the horrors of camping and using festival toilets in the middle of the night. We love going to the music festivals, and if we couldn't see Matt play, then we would set our souls free in the sunshine and join the beautiful people at Seaclose Park. We had to interrupt this idyll as we had been invited to attend Anna's brother Alex's wedding on the Saturday in Sudbury, but it was back on the ferry Saturday night to see The Police close the festival on the Sunday evening.

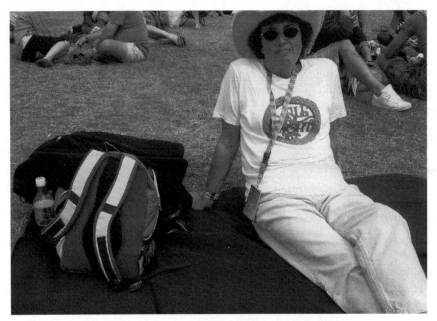

Myself at the Isle of Wight Festival June 2008

An unexpected bonus occurred in July. Phil booked a surprise weekend trip to Dublin for us. We flew from Stansted airport and stayed in the Temple Bar area. I dragged him around St. Fintan's graveyard looking for Thin Lizzy frontman Phil Lynott's grave (we found it after a long search), visited Oscar Wilde's house in Merrion Square, and enjoyed a Riverdance performance at the Gaiety Theatre. What a lovely weekend. There were walks along the banks of the Liffey, and also shopping in the famous Grafton Street. All too soon it came to an end, and it was back to work again on Monday.

Two family birthdays occurred in July. Granddaughter Sophie was three, and our eldest son Lee was 26. Lee was now a Service Manager - no longer the air-conditioning apprentice doomed forever to make the tea and get the bacon torpedoes in. He has made a name for himself in the air-conditioning industry as one of the best Engineers around. Matt at the tender age of 22 has recently been promoted to Supervisor in his field as a CNC Machine Programmer. I was very proud of my ever-growing family, and wanted to be around for quite a few more years to see my granddaughters grow up.

CHAPTER TWENTY-SIX – ONE YEAR AFTER THE NECK DISSECTION

We had been invited to another wedding in August 2008. Mary and Dave's eldest daughter Clare was marrying her long-term partner Steve. She looked stunning in her dress on the day, and it was lovely to have all the family together and happy. I do like weddings. Unfortunately Lee and Sarah couldn't make the wedding, but Matt and Anna turned up for the evening reception and we danced the night away.

My youngest granddaughter Caitlin was one on August 14th, and Sarah organised a little party for her. The Monday following the party I was back at the Nuffield in Cambridge to see the Oncologist for a check-up.

The Oncologist was all smiles after she had felt around my neck, and assured me that my neck felt 'perfectly normal'. Thank goodness for that. She booked me in for a scan in December, and I had some blood taken to check for thyroglobulin levels, TSH, T3, and T4. She made an appointment for me to see her again on December 8th to get the results of the latest CT scan. All seemed well. The last blood test done a couple of weeks before at the GP surgery showed my eosinophil count had gone down to 1.3, so at the moment all was groovy in my little world.

About a month after the blood test, the results came in. My thyroglobulin levels had reduced to 0.5, thyroglobulin antibodies had reduced to just under 500 (they had been near to 1000 the previous year), and TSH was less than 0.03. The neck dissection had been worth it. These results were all encouraging. The only downside was that my T4 level was 32 – too high! I would have to reduce my Thyroxine dosage slightly. The Oncologist suggested taking 125mcg of Thyroxine on Mondays, Wednesdays, and Fridays, and 150mcg the rest of the week. There would be another blood test nearer Christmas when my scan was due to check if this new dose was right for me. I hoped I would not start putting on weight with the reduced dose, as up till now I had been able to eat what I wanted and still stay the same weight. However, if I had to have an operation where I had to be nil by mouth for a day, then I could lose half a stone in a day. Perhaps the Thyroxine dose was slightly too high for me!

Whilst I had been waiting for the blood test results, something very unexpected happened. Matthew and Anna announced their engagement on September 3rd. They had been together for 6 years, so I suppose it was about time! I envisioned Anna's Mum and I having fun organising a big engagement party for them, and there would be another family wedding to look forward to in 2010. The setting had been quite romantic for the proposal. Matt had popped the question whilst they were on holiday with Anna's family in Canada. They were staying at her auntie's cottage on Bruce Beach, and he had waited until it was sunset and then had got down on one knee on the beach with a lovely engagement ring in his hand. Ah! Needless to say Anna said 'yes'! I now had two sons, two daughters –in-law, two granddaughters, one very lovely husband, and good blood results. What more could I want? My cup was running over as they say. To cap it all I had received a 'normal' result from my first routine mammogram which all women over 50 are encouraged to have, and another above average score for my age on a further bone density scan. It was nice to be 'normal' for a change.

There was also a break in Beaulieu Sur Dordogne, France, at the end of September. We had been invited to stay with the Managing Director of the company where Phil works and his wife in their house for a long weekend. After knowing them for over 20 years they were more like friends than employer and employee. They paid for our airfare, met us at the airport, and showed us the sights around their local area. Their house was more like a mansion, and boasted a large swimming pool, a cinema room, a bar and wine cellar, a pool/snooker room, and in fact anything you could possibly want. The weather was gorgeous for the end of summer, and we swam in the pool every day and ate from the barbeque on the large patio at night. We visited the huge market at Salat, the village and chapel carved from the rocks at Rocamadour, and a restaurant with stunning views over the valley and Dordogne river at Domme. At the end of our visit they took us back to the airport, making sure we had some lunch with us! What more could you want from your employers!

October 2008 saw me back at the GP surgery for a NHS re-referral to the Eye Clinic at the hospital where I work. No matter how I tried to stick to the instructions given to me the last time I attended when it was thought I had blepharitis, it made no difference. My eyes still became infected, sore and watery on now increasingly regular occasions, and I was becoming very tired of constantly having to wipe my watery eyes all the time. My eyes were also over-sensitive to light, causing me to always have to wear dark glasses when outside, and I always tried to avoid driving at night due to other cars' headlights being too dazzling. The GP informed me that patients with thyroid problems always seem to have eye problems as well, but he agreed with the Ophthalmologist's last letter when he remarked that he thought my problems had nothing whatsoever to do with having three doses of radiation. He prescribed Chloramphenicol ointment, which unfortunately did not work. I wondered how was it then that my eye problems only started after having the RAI treatment? An appointment was sent to me to attend the Eye Clinic on November 17th.

I mentioned the eye problem to my mother a few weeks before I was due to attend the clinic. She came up with the old-fashioned remedy of cleaning the eyes with a solution of Sodium Bicarbonate twice a day (a quarter of a teaspoon in cooled, boiled water). I tried that and it worked to start with, but found I still had eye infections from time to time, and my eyes still watered when I walked outside in a cold wind. Nothing really seemed to work. Another visit to a different GP ensued before the Eye Clinic appointment. This GP suggested using some baby shampoo in warm water and cotton buds to scrub the eyelids every day, as she was sure it was blepharitis. She also took a swab, as I had an eye infection at the time. I trawled the internet in desperation and found a correlation between cumulative doses of RAI and a blockage of the eyes' drainage systems causing watery eyes and frequent conjunctivitis. Result! The condition is called epiphora, and I had all the symptoms.

If it was found that I had this problem, then it could be cured with minor surgery. I would mention it at the Eye Clinic appointment.

The last of my three healing appointments occurred at the end of October. The Healer informed me that I was 'as fit as a fiddle' and there was 'nothing wrong with me'. I had just bought two of his books and was reading about his childhood experiences with psychic phenomena, so I hoped he knew what he was talking about. He had also experienced his bed moving as a young child, and I felt an affinity with him as I turned the pages (people do tend to look at you strangely when you mention something like this!). He did not ask me to make another appointment, but I said I might be in touch after my scan results in December (I like to keep my options open) if I wasn't given the all clear.

There was another successful check-up with the ENT Surgeon on 10th November. He placed the well-hated scope in the right nostril again to check on the vocal cords and the back of the throat (my heart sinks when I see that scope). I had mentioned to him that very occasionally (about five times a year) food or phlegm would get stuck at the back of my throat making it difficult for me to breathe in, and I would have to cough very hard to dislodge it. To me it seemed as though my windpipe was blocked when this happened. He reassured me that the paralysed vocal cord was in quite a good position, and the back of my throat looked normal. Because of its position, there was not much that could be done to move the vocal cord to a position where the strength of my voice could be improved and to stop the windpipe being occasionally blocked. There was a risk that any operation performed could also make me permanently short of breath, with no real relief of symptoms. I told him I'd leave it. I realised this was the 'new normal' and I would have to live with it. He could feel no new lumps in my neck though, and said he didn't need to see me again for six months. He said he would meet up with the Oncologist to have a look at the CT scan which I was to have on 5th December. If any more enlarged lymph nodes showed up, he informed me that he could operate and remove them.

By now the effects of the reduced dose of Thyroxine were beginning to kick in. I found I did not feel as hot as before, but unfortunately I had put on half a stone in weight. The temptation was to buy bigger trousers, but if I did that I would just be buying bigger and bigger ones as time went by, so I decided to cut down a bit on the Mr Kipling lemon slices, which fortunately never seemed to block my windpipe however many of them I ate.

At the end of November there was a lovely party at Abington Hall, Cambridge, to celebrate Matt and Anna's engagement. We danced all night, and met up with Mary and Dave, and Phil's nieces Clare, with new husband Steve, and Jenny with her boyfriend, and nephew Paul. Matt and Anna had organised everything themselves including the music and a slideshow of old photos of them as babies. Lee and Sarah came along (having secured a babysitter at the last minute), and it was lovely to have all the family together.

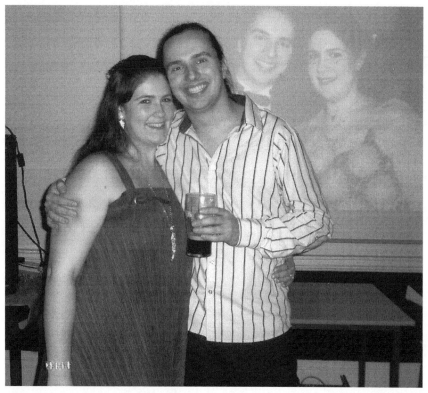

Matt and Anna at their engagement party – November 29th 2008.

The dreaded appointment with the Oncologist came on the 8th December 2008 to get the results of a CT scan I had had three days previously. Walking into her office that morning after having no sleep for three nights due to worrying about what might be found, I was not feeling at my best. I had taken heart though from all the good wishes on Facebook from my family and friends, and was trying to think positively. The Oncologist was quick to point out that nothing had changed since the last scan; the tiny lung spots were still there but had not grown due to their growth being suppressed with Thyroxine, and the two slightly enlarged lymph glands in my neck that the ENT Surgeon had mentioned after my previous scan a year before had not enlarged either, and were unchanged. The Oncologist did also say that the two lymph glands might just be slightly enlarged anyway in their normal state, and possibly were not cancerous at all. As far as she could tell, I was in remission. All I needed was a blood test to check that my new Thyroxine level was correct. I had mentioned the slight weight gain, but Phil and I picked up on the overall vibes that if the levels were correct I would just have to eat less (the gates of heaven are narrow I hear, and if I eat too many lemon slices I will not be able to get in when the time comes).

Such a relief! I was in remission! I had been waiting a long time to hear this. I had been given a new lease of life, and I was going to make the most of it. Phil and I walked back to the car that morning on cloud nine.

Also after mentioning my frequent eye infections and watery eyes to the Oncologist, she sent an urgent faxed referral to a Consultant Ophthalmologist at the Nuffield hospital in Bury, and I would receive an appointment to see him two days later. I cancelled the NHS Eye Clinic appointment, as I knew it would be better to see a Consultant, and I would not necessarily have seen one at my NHS appointment.

When the blood test result came back, it showed that the thyroid stimulating hormone level was raised too much. If I carried on with the reduced Thyroxine dose, then probably the lung spots would start to grow. The Oncologist quickly sent me instructions to go back to the original dose of 150mcg. There was an upside to this news though - I could now put Mr Kipling's lemon slices back on my weekly shopping list. Some more good news; the thyroglobulin level eventually came back as less than 0.5, and the thyroglobulin antibodies had reduced even more from September and were now 441.4.

Back at the Nuffield again for my eye appointment, the Ophthalmologist measured the pressure in each eye (which was normal), and applied some yellow dye to check if the tear ducts were working – they were. He diagnosed recurrent follicular conjunctivitis, which he said was a non-bacterial infection probably caused by the radiation. It was the frequent infections that were making the tear ducts swollen and therefore narrower. He prescribed some steroid eye drops for me to take for two months to see if they stopped the infections. He told me not to use baby shampoo to clean the eyes with, but to stick to the Sodium Bicarbonate solution. I was to see him again for review after the two months were up. If the steroid did not work, then he would try something else. At last it looked as if the eye problems would soon be sorted out as well. What a wonderful Christmas it was going to be this year!

CHAPTER 27 - EPILOGUE

So, after two major operations, three doses of radiation, and four years on from finding the original lump, how am I today? Because I have only one vocal cord I have a weak voice that is fine for day to day living, but put me in a room with loud music or loud background noise and I will struggle to make myself heard. I cannot read long passages aloud to my grandchildren without gasping for breath, and I cannot sing a song all the way through, as I cannot seem to breathe in fast enough to keep up, and also can't reach high notes. I am 'lucky' in that I did not have this affliction when my boys were small, as some degree of shouting had to be undertaken on my part on quite a frequent basis (the ENT Surgeon does tell me though, that compared to his other patients with the same condition, my voice is one of the better ones). Also again probably because of the paralysed cord food very occasionally becomes stuck in the back of my throat, making it rather alarming for fellow diners if I am out in a restaurant when this occurs. If I have a cold or cough, my voice is the first thing I lose and it is the last thing to return once the germ goes away. There is still a slight phlegm problem caused by the uptake of RAI at the back of my throat, which occurred during my last stay in Addenbrooke's RAI suite in November 2006, but it is slowly improving. My left jaw joint is not very robust and I have to avoid biting down on hard foodstuffs, but it does not lock any more. On a happier note, my eyes haven't been as watery or infected since starting the steroid drops, so hopefully this problem will soon ease. The left side of my neck and top of my left shoulder remain numb, and probably always will be, and oh yes, I don't do heat. Due to all that extra Thyroxine pumping round, my body temperature is higher than everyone else's and I am hot quite a lot of the time. After living with me for nearly 30 years, Phil doesn't do heat either, and our visitors usually know to put extra jumpers on when they visit. Our faces are always redder than anyone else's, we haven't got central heating, and couldn't think of anything worse than having to sit in a hot, stuffy room. We actually have an air-conditioning unit in our lounge instead (thanks Lee!), and cooling fans in every room that get used a lot in the summer months.

But hey, there are millions of people worse off than me. Working as a Medical Secretary and typing clinic letters for other people tells me that, and I am grateful to still be here to see my granddaughters growing up. I am looking forward to our cruise aboard the Royal Caribbean's ship 'Radiance of the Seas' in February 2009 which will visit various ports in South America and also stop for us to attend the Rio de Janeiro carnival, and I still aim to be around on 6th August 2010 for Matt and Anna's wedding day. Anna asked me to write a poem to be read on their special day, and I have included it below (only because they have already read it and approve!). I will ask Anna's brother Alex to read it out on the day, as the problems I have would make it impossible for me to project my voice across a large room.

Here's to good health!

TO MATT AND ANNA ON THEIR WEDDING DAY

1   Two brown soulful eyes,
A wise little face,
A new brother for Lee,
I look at Matthew
And he looks at me.

2   He's quiet and shy,
Where I go
There he'll be,
I cuddle Matthew
And he cuddles me.

3   Not keen on playgroup,
Doesn't want to learn,
Two sad brown eyes
Await my return.

4   First day at school
He's grown so tall,
He's made me a picture
To hang on the wall.

5   Now he goes to Upper school,
Runs for the bus so as not to be late,
Waves goodbye at the garden gate.
He visits friends who live near and far,
One day he sees my old guitar.

6   "Teach me some chords Mum",
        The guitar's in his hand,
        Before you know it,
        He's joined a band.

7   He grows his hair
        His friends aren't posh,
        Some of them
        Don't appear to ever wash.

8   "We need a Singer"
        Who will it be?
        I place some adverts.
        We wait and see.

9   A girl replies,
        She sends a text.
        They arrange to meet
        On Saturday next.

10   She arrives in a car
        With her Father and Mother,
        They've both come to see
        Who's got his eye on their daughter.

11   Her Father jumps out
        Shakes Matt by the hand,
        Her Mother's less keen,
        Anna's only fifteen.

12   Matt has long hair, big boots,
        A leather jacket and all,
        Alison's phone is by her ear
        In case Anna has to call.

13   They walk and talk,
The time flies by,
Now Anna meets us
Who are waiting nearby.

14   They walk towards us
Hand in hand,
That's quick work thinks I,
It pays to be in a band.

15   She's a very sweet girl
With long dark hair,
She answered the advert
For a dare.

16   My son is in love
The world around him grows dim.
He cuddles Anna,
And she cuddles him.

17   And so it must pass,
It's part of nature's plan,
From mother to wife,
Now he's grown to a man.

18   As we sit here today,
I'll say to each and every one,
I've gained a daughter,
Not lost a son.

About the Author

I live in a rather picturesque village near Bury St Edmunds in Suffolk, U.K, and work as a Medical Secretary. I have been married to Phil for 28 years, and have two grown-up sons and two granddaughters. My interests include attending music festivals and concerts, reading autobiographies, and I enjoy going to the gym and walking in the countryside to keep fit.